CROHN'S DISEASE AIP COOKBOOK

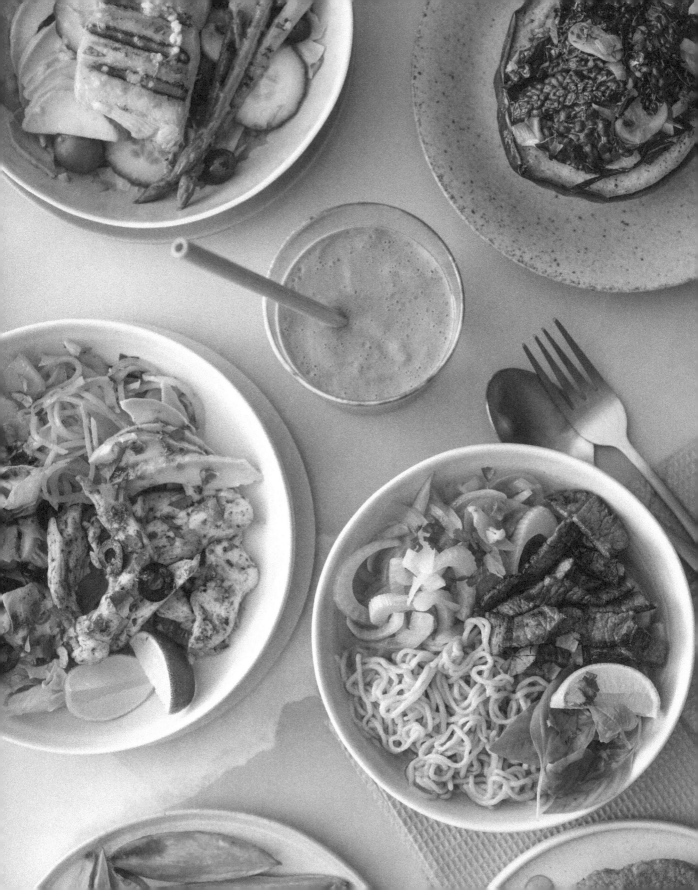

CROHN'S DISEASE AIP COOKBOOK

Recipes to Reduce Inflammation and Eliminate Food Triggers on the Autoimmune Protocol

JOSHUA BRADLEY AND KIA SANFORD, MS

PHOTOGRAPHY BY DARREN MUIR

ROCKRIDGE
PRESS

Copyright © 2022 by Rockridge Press, Oakland, California

For general information on our other products and services or to obtain technical support, please contact our Customer Care Department within the United States at (866) 744-2665, or outside the United States at (510) 253-0500.

Rockridge Press publishes its books in a variety of electronic and print formats. Some content that appears in print may not be available in electronic books, and vice versa.

Interior and Cover Designer: Stephanie Sumulong
Art Producer: Maya Melenchuk
Editor: Owen Holmes
Production Manager: Riley Hoffman

Photography © 2022 Darren Muir

Paperback ISBN: 978-1-63878-040-3 | eBook ISBN: 978-1-63878-763-1
R0

*For Amanda and
my Frazley girls, always.
—Joshua*

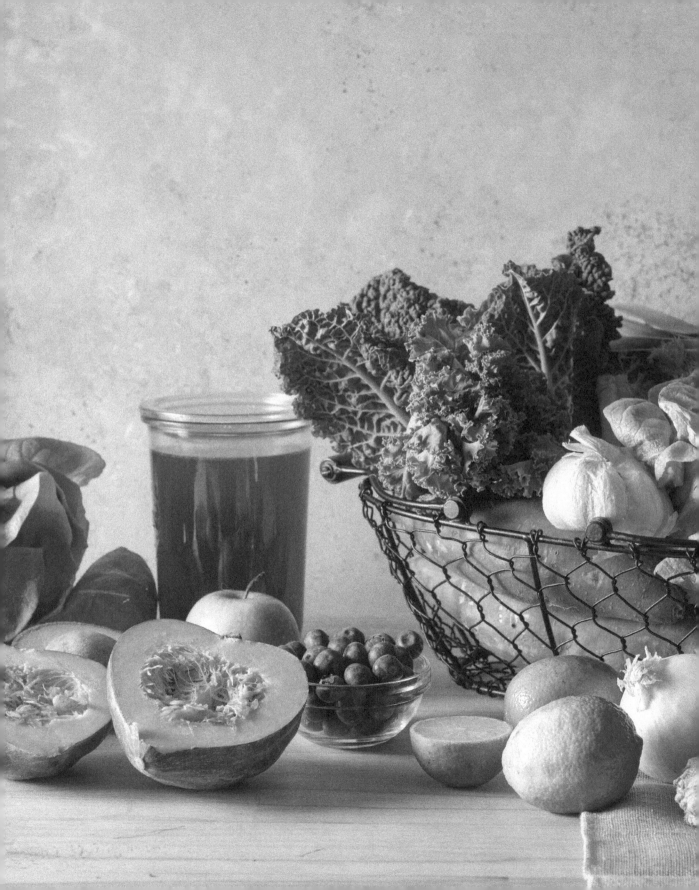

Contents

Introduction

A Few Words from Joshua: In my own way, I've been where you are now. I was diagnosed with Crohn's disease in 2013 after losing 90 pounds in three months. When the test confirming inflammatory bowel disease (IBD) came back, my inflammation levels were so high that a representative for the lab went to my doctor's office to see if I was a real person. Within a year, I underwent emergency surgery after discovering an abscess the size of a softball and several fistulas, a potential complication of Crohn's with high inflammation. Although I'm not a medical professional or a nutritionist, I spent the subsequent eight years getting a veritable PhD in myself and have enjoyed the last three years in deep remission thanks to thousands of hours of my own research and experimentation, and the help and guidance of a team of doctors, surgeons, and my coauthor for this book, Kia.

A key psychological shift in my recovery came from discovering *SuperBetter*, Jane McGonigal's book about "gamifying" her recovery from a head injury. Making my health journey into a game, I went from no exercise to riding a single-speed bicycle in a 50-mile Gran Fondo, a type of long-distance road-cycling ride. I've since suffered through numerous surgeries, but I've also ridden my bike from San Francisco to Los Angeles with the AIDS/LifeCycle foundation and trained to swim and run to compete in the Hope for Crohn's triathlon. In 2021, I ran my first half-marathon.

Having IBD makes food feel like an impossible puzzle. To sustain my training, I had to figure out how to generate energy while sick. The autoimmune protocol (AIP) helped reduce my symptoms, and intermittent fasting minimized the amount of time my body spent digesting, increasing the time spent healing. Having worked as a fine dining chef, I applied my understanding of cooking techniques to produce delicious and nutrient-dense food. Thinking of your disease and diet as a journey that is unfolding—rather than a destination to arrive at—will make you open to recognizing and appreciating progress.

A Few Words from Kia: As a clinical nutritionist, I work with many people who are struggling with complex illnesses, such as IBD, that often stump conventional medicine. To make matters more complicated, no two bodies manifest IBD the same way. To maximize your chances of full remission, it is important to have someone who is well versed in nutritional approaches to IBD on your team to be sure you get the nutrients your body needs to heal and to mitigate the side effects of the medications you may have to take. This is Joshua's story, and we hope it will help you navigate your situation, but understand that your needs may be different.

Chapters 1 and 2 of this book introduce the autoimmune protocol and how you can use it to manage Crohn's symptoms and discover potential irritants. Chapters 3 through 9 provide 76 AIP-compliant recipes for all types of meals during the elimination phase of the AIP diet. These recipes can also be used throughout reintroduction as you move to a less-restrictive diet. Our goal is to not only help you cook food in your home using common ingredients but also change how you look at food. We hope you'll find recipes in your exploration that become favorites.

The back of the book contains several resources, including a guide to reintroducing foods and how to track symptoms for trigger foods. This book is not intended to be an exhaustive list of every potential dietary issue, so be sure to consult with your doctor and/or nutritionist for dietary guidance.

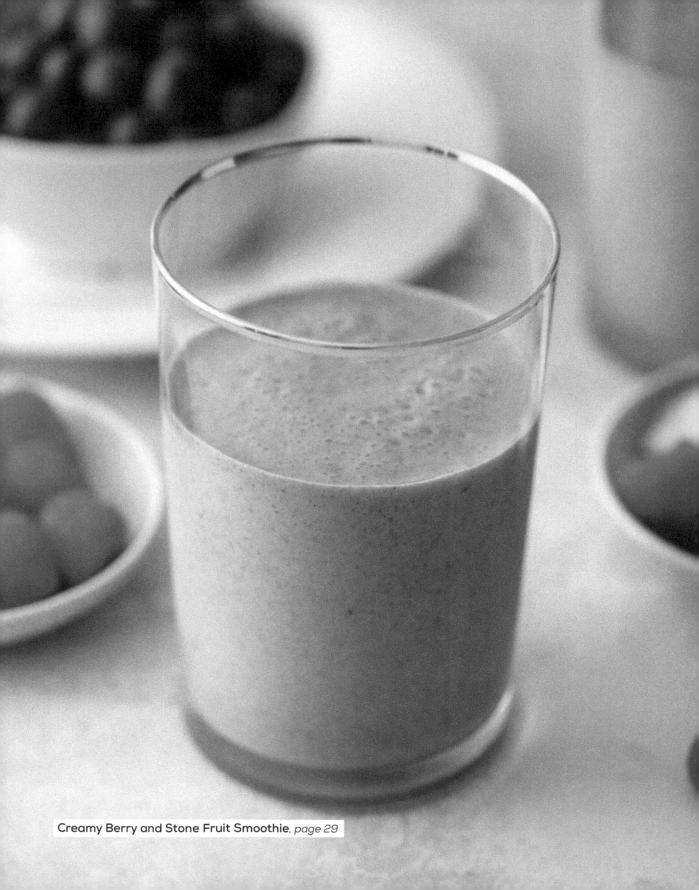

Creamy Berry and Stone Fruit Smoothie, *page 29*

CHAPTER 1

MANAGING CROHN'S WITH THE AIP

In this chapter, we discuss inflammatory bowel disease (IBD), the difference between ulcerative colitis and Crohn's disease, and the relationship between diet and lifestyle. We will also outline the autoimmune protocol (AIP) and how to use it to get to a baseline that allows you to pinpoint potential trigger foods.

Defining Crohn's Disease

Crohn's disease is an autoimmune disorder and one of two inflammatory bowel diseases characterized by chronic inflammation and damage in the gastrointestinal tract (the other being ulcerative colitis). Autoimmune disease makes your body mistakenly attack its own cells. The difference between Crohn's and ulcerative colitis is that the latter causes inflammation confined to the large intestine, whereas Crohn's disease can manifest anywhere in the digestive tract. This can make Crohn's flare-ups quite painful, exhibiting as anything from mouth sores to ulcerations in the small intestine or large bowel. The dietary approach outlined in this book can be useful in both types of IBD.

Weight loss due to frequent visits to the bathroom is easy to understand, but having such extreme chronic inflammation makes it difficult for your body to absorb nutrients, which can cause several additional issues ranging from skin problems to fatigue to trouble building muscle mass. This constellation of symptoms, combined with a complex relationship to food that may make symptoms worse, makes communicating the experience of having Crohn's to other people difficult and uncomfortable.

Although there is no cure for IBD, rest assured that there are ways to achieve long-term health goals in which life feels normal. Remission is possible, and you may someday find yourself healthier overall than you were before your symptoms began. IBD is caused by a number of contributing factors, from environmental triggers to genetics to lifestyle choices. Going through this journey of healing can lead you to create a life that aligns with achieving and maintaining health.

That has certainly been Joshua's experience. Despite having a colostomy and surgeries that changed his life forever, deep remission has allowed him to create a life with stronger relationships, become a better father, and achieve athletic accomplishments he never dreamed possible. With this book, he hopes you gain an understanding of how to eat to thrive while developing a lifestyle and a long-term path toward remission.

Understanding the Connection between Crohn's and Diet

There are several dietary approaches that can be effectively used to improve symptoms related to Crohn's, but there is no specific IBD diet. You may have heard of (or tried) the GAPS, low FODMAP, low residue, or even the carnivore diet to find relief, and depending on the individual disease state, any of these can be effective. Because Crohn's is an autoimmune disease, dietary choices can worsen disease severity if foods trigger an overactive immune response, which can make diets difficult. Discovering your food triggers is an essential part of the AIP approach. You do this by first eliminating most foods known to irritate and cause inflammation, then slowly reintroducing foods to pinpoint your triggers. Part of the difficulty is that everyone's body reacts differently to food. Your triggers might not be the same as someone else's, even if you both have Crohn's. It is important to have an open mind and be flexible about your diet from day to day, as well as during different times in your life, based on how you're feeling and your disease activity.

The Importance of Nutrition

While in a state of chronic inflammation, the body cannot absorb nutrients in the same way it does when it is healthy. To further complicate matters, nutrients are absorbed by the small intestine, which may have spots of damaged lining. Micro bleeding from the damage inside your gastrointestinal tract can also cause low iron or anemia. Although it may seem as though your whole body is working against you, being diligent about your nutrition is one of the ways you can work to improve digestion and absorption.

Having Crohn's, you need to be sure to get enough calories from the right food sources. Additionally, other aspects of eating, such as slowing down the speed at which you eat, can provide significant help to your impaired digestion. The ability to maintain a healthy weight (and even healthy hair, skin, and nails) is a strong signal that the body is getting enough nutrients and using them appropriately.

Because digestion and absorption are compromised by Crohn's, supplements are sometimes needed to make sure that our bodies have enough building blocks. It is vital to get adequate amounts of vitamins D and K, B vitamins such as folate, and vitamins A and E. Minerals such as zinc, magnesium, potassium, and calcium are important for tissue repair, blood cell production, and neurological health. Omega-3 fatty acids can be hugely beneficial to people with Crohn's, because they are powerful anti-inflammatories that have been shown to reduce inflammation in the walls of the intestine. We highly recommend a high-quality omega-3 or fish oil supplement.

You have likely heard a lot about probiotics, and there are specific strains that have been identified as being beneficial for people with Crohn's, but prebiotic fiber is key to establishing viable colonies of the good guys. Fiber can be a controversial subject in dealing with Crohn's. During flare-ups, any fiber can cause issues such as gas, bloating, and even increased diarrhea. But fiber is important to building and maintaining a healthy gut. There are two types of fiber: soluble and insoluble.

Soluble fiber creates a sponge-like gel when dissolved in water and may be useful in helping take up some of the extra fluid in the gut to slow digestion and provide some relief from diarrhea. Beneficial soluble fiber can be found in foods such as avocados, apples, chia seeds, Brussels sprouts, carrots, sweet potatoes, green beans, and squash.

Insoluble fiber acts like a scrubber as it passes along the GI tract. Too much insoluble fiber may make symptoms worse, increasing gas, stomach cramps, and diarrhea. Insoluble fiber foods include leafy greens, broccoli, whole grains, nuts and seeds, and the skins of many fruits and vegetables. We strive to get the right balance of fiber while following the AIP.

A NOTE ON SUPPLEMENTS FROM KIA

It's important to understand that nutritional supplements are supposed to *supplement* a meal plan that covers a person's nutrient needs as completely as possible, not replace food or "fix" a diet made of nutrient-poor choices. In IBD, digestion and absorption of nutrients from food are often compromised, and supplementation becomes essential. Some supplement companies hold to ideals of providing the highest-quality and most-bioavailable nutrients available, but many put profits before quality. It is extremely important to work with a qualified professional to help you find supplements that will work for your situation. Nutrient forms, base material sourcing, processing mechanisms, delivery method, and proper dosing all matter greatly.

There are a few nutrients I can recommend to most people struggling with IBD because I've seen so many clients suffering from depletions of these nutrients. Consult a nutritionist well-versed in IBD about oil-based vitamin D_3, glutathione, N-acetylcysteine (NAC), eicosapentaenoic acid (EPA), zinc carnosine, methyl-folate, and nonhistamine-producing probiotics, which can be beneficial for healing the mucosal lining, reducing inflammation, and stemming symptom progression.

As always, discuss all supplements with a medical professional first before adding them to your diet.

Autoimmune Protocol (AIP) Explained

The AIP is an elimination diet in which potentially problematic foods are removed to reduce digestive symptoms, as well as to get a sense of what may or may not be contributing to those symptoms. After a period of elimination, foods are reintroduced methodically to identify problem foods that may need to be avoided at that time.

Autoimmunity is when the immune system, which is designed to produce antibodies to attack harmful invaders, mistakenly turns on healthy cells. Many medical professionals believe that most, if not all, autoimmune disorders start with some form of gut dysfunction, commonly described as *leaky gut*. Certain foods are believed to increase gut permeability, allowing incompletely digested food particles and toxins to cross the gut barrier, causing the immune system to react to what it perceives as foreign invaders. The AIP is focused on eliminating foods associated with the inflammation response and healing gut hyperpermeability with nutrient-dense foods that support the gut lining.

One of the main foods to eliminate that can cause a lot of anxiety for people is gluten, which is found in wheat and other types of grains. There is research showing that a component of gluten called *gliadin* opens the tight junctions between the mucosal cells of the gut lining, creating a leaky gut by releasing a substance called *zonulin*. The problem may even be worse for people with certain genetic variants.

The AIP has two phases: First, inflammatory foods are eliminated; then, once symptoms stabilize, foods or food groups are slowly reintroduced to help get a sense of what is causing or contributing to symptoms.

Elimination Phase

During the elimination phase, grains, legumes, nuts, seeds, nightshades, eggs, and dairy are removed completely. It is also important to avoid coffee, alcohol, refined oils, processed sugars, and food additives, as well as all nonsteroidal anti-inflammatory drugs (NSAIDs), including ibuprofen and low-dose aspirin (make sure you discuss the elimination of any medications with your doctor before stopping).

Nightshades are a family of plants that includes tomatoes, potatoes, eggplants, bell peppers and chiles, and goji berries. These plants produce irritating alkaloids that function as natural pesticides as they grow. Some people are more sensitive than others, but nightshades are to be avoided during the elimination phase.

This approach feels very restrictive relative to a standard diet, but although there are a lot of things that you can't eat on the AIP during the elimination phase, there are many foods you can eat to create delicious meals. It is important to note that the AIP is not a weight-loss diet, so you shouldn't be concerned with calories as much as how the food makes you feel and what your energy levels are like. Such a dramatic shift in diet is likely to feel different (hopefully providing some swift relief!), but you shouldn't feel as though you aren't getting enough nourishment. The goal is to increase nutrient uptake while eliminating foods that can cause inflammation or irritation to the gut lining.

The good news is you can eat nearly any kind of fish or meat, as well as all non-nightshade vegetables and most fruits with the skin removed. We promise you are going to find recipes in this book that are as—or even more—delicious than anything you've cooked before. We are going to boost nutrients with the richness from bone broth and introduce healthy fats, such as coconut and avocado, to provide long-lasting fuel for energizing your cells.

After completing the elimination phase, which typically lasts for 30 to 90 days depending on symptoms, you will start to reintroduce foods. There is a complete list of foods that are part of the elimination phase in chapter 2 of this book.

Reintroduction Phase

During the second phase of the AIP, foods or food groups are reintroduced one at a time, with the goal of identifying which ones contribute to symptoms. Before you start the reintroduction phase, you should be feeling a dramatic reduction in symptoms. If you aren't feeling better, reintroducing foods would make it difficult to know which foods might be causing a problem. This stage is about rebuilding your regular diet in a way that serves your health. Start by introducing one food or food group for

PINPOINTING YOUR FOOD TRIGGERS

Each person is unique—as is the severity of each person's disease state. What causes symptoms for one person may be tolerated just fine by someone else. Similarly, at different times of your life and in different points in your health, the foods that may cause or trigger symptoms may be totally different.

We've included a symptom tracker at the end of this book (page 139) that will help you monitor your Crohn's disease response as you reintroduce foods. Keeping track of your food intake is important to the success of evaluating what is helping and what is hurting. During reintroduction, you will be adding foods methodically and eating them daily to get a true sense of how you feel. If you try to rely solely on memory, all the hard work done in the elimination phase will be lost.

Joshua, for example, has kept a symptom tracker for six years, and it has allowed him to look back to any period and match up what he was eating and feeling at that time. A food log during times of feeling good is basically a blueprint for eating what he knows can work for him and understanding reactions to food in the present by looking at his history.

a period of five to seven days to gauge how it feels and whether the addition causes symptoms.

Ideally, reintroduction goes slowly, one to two months at a time, starting with foods based on nutrient density and known impact on inflammation. Many of these foods would be considered healthy, so it is important not to look at them as bad or good but rather what is working for you right now and what is not. For example, dairy and eggs are two of the most common triggers, but they are also rich in nutrients and are used to make many tasty meals. You may choose to start there.

However, if you react to one food or food group during the reintroduction phase, it doesn't mean you have to cut it out forever. Remember, your body is healing from a chronic alarm state and leaks in the gut lining. Wait until things are sufficiently stable before reintroducing reactionary foods again.

There is a guide at the back of the book called How to Reintroduce Foods (page 136) that will give you guidelines on how to properly reintroduce foods. The recipes in this book are intended to support you during the reintroduction phase and can be modified to include reintroduced ingredients. We hope you find new favorites you can bring with you as you come to the end of your AIP journey.

How the AIP Works with Crohn's Disease

As we've discussed, Crohn's and ulcerative colitis are two types of IBD. They each have distinct disease patterns, but they are treated similarly by conventional therapies. Most commonly, pharmaceuticals designed to suppress the immune system are prescribed. These medications have a huge variation in efficacy from person to person, often with debilitating side effects. Despite it being widely acknowledged that autoimmunity begins in the gut, many gastroenterologists don't recognize diet and lifestyle as significant avenues for relief from this incredibly disruptive and painful disease.

The 2017 study published in *Inflammatory Bowel Diseases* showed how dietary elimination can improve both reported symptoms (how people felt) and measured inflammation levels. The study successfully pulled the curtain back on the complexity of IBD, showing that it is highly affected by environmental factors, including dysfunctional cellular health, gut dysbiosis (an imbalance in the bacterial and fungal populations of the gut), and diet.

The AIP was born out of the Paleo diet, adding a methodical approach to eliminating foods known as potential gut irritants and inflammation contributors to what has commonly been called *leaky gut*. The elimination period is followed by a maintenance phase intended to expand available food options as symptoms and well-being improve, while catching foods that contribute to symptoms.

The AIP is used as an intervention diet, but we are using it as a diagnostic tool that quiets the noise introduced by inflammation so that you can more clearly access the signals of healing. In the 2017 study mentioned earlier, 73 percent of participants achieved clinical remission after the initial six-week phase, which continued during the maintenance phase for all participants. The AIP has been successful for people with Crohn's in stopping what can feel like a free fall and offering a pathway to understanding how environmental factors, such as diet and lifestyle, can work as a force for health and not just illness.

Eating for the Long-Term

You've finished the elimination phase and reintroduced foods to determine which foods are causing triggers, and you've started building a stable diet that works for your life. Unfortunately, this doesn't mean everything will remain the same forever—you may have flare-ups, and new foods may cause other symptoms. You may be able to tolerate one or two trigger foods per day but not three, or you may only be able to tolerate a few tablespoons of a certain food at a time. Having gone through this protocol, you now have a baseline to return to. You can use it to eliminate the foods that you discovered were triggers.

If needed, you can return to the AIP and start the cycle over again until the symptoms go away, and you'll have more information about what works and what doesn't. The recipes in this book can be eaten at any time and are based on many of Joshua's favorite foods. Our families approve of their deliciousness and request several on a regular basis. We hope you enjoy them as well and that they help fuel a healthy and happy future.

FOOD FOR FLARE-UPS

Eating during flare-ups can be difficult. Often you just want to eat what makes you feel good. Unfortunately, what feels comforting may not actually provide the nutrients the body needs, or worse, it may contribute to Crohn's symptoms. The AIP should help remove most or all of the foods that can induce inflammation and trigger a flare-up, but there are several foods you can keep on hand that are both nutritious and gentle on the body when flare-ups happen. Here are Joshua's top 10 foods to eat during a flare-up:

1. Applesauce (unsweetened)
2. Fatty, omega-3-rich fish, such as salmon, sardines, and mackerel
3. Bone broth
4. Sweet potatoes (no skin)
5. Avocados
6. Soft, fleshy fruits (no skin or seeds)
7. Lean meats
8. Bananas or plantains
9. Cassava (never eat raw)
10. Cultured coconut yogurt

Joshua's number one food hack for inflammation is Applesauce (page 110) cooked with the skins all the way down so that all the pectin gets released, and then blended with a little bit of cinnamon. The pectin from whole apples has been shown to have a powerful anti-inflammatory benefit, including reducing CRP (C-reactive protein) by 32 percent, according to a study published in *Critical Reviews in Food Science and Nutrition*.

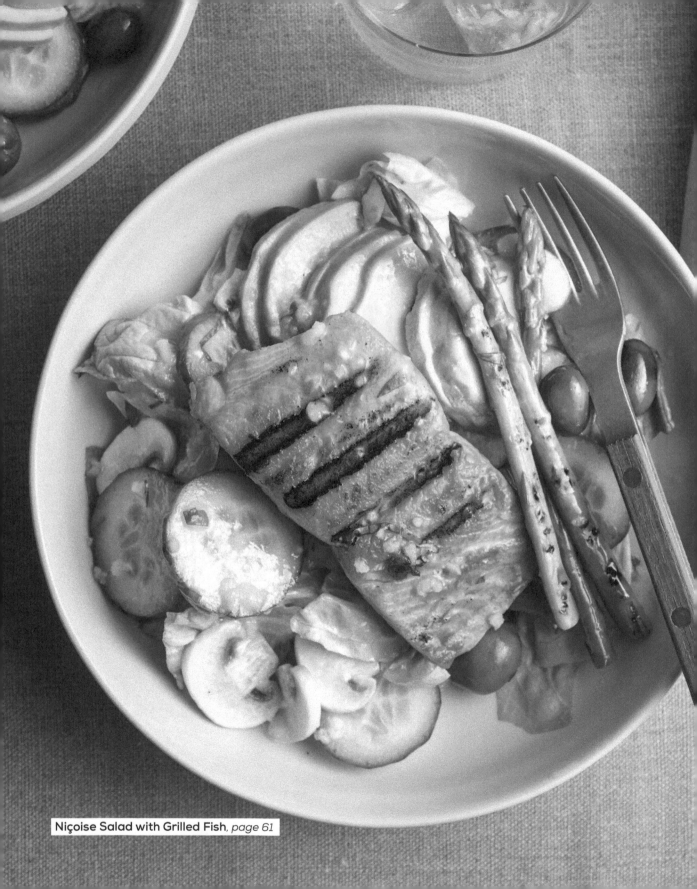

Niçoise Salad with Grilled Fish, *page 61*

CHAPTER 2

THE AIP KITCHEN AND SAMPLE MEAL PLAN

In this chapter, we help you transform your pantry for the next couple of months. We'll lay out what to avoid and, more important, what you can enjoy. We also include a sample meal plan and tips to make it easy to integrate the AIP into your life.

Foods to Enjoy on the AIP

Let's start with the foods you can enjoy freely, without worrying about things like serving sizes or food categories. The foods in this section are rich in antioxidants, plant-based fiber, and healthy fats to keep you going. If you have a farmers' market nearby, go weekly. It's a great habit that helps you not only acquire high-quality ingredients but also relax into a routine that can be shared with family and friends.

If you don't have a farmers' market, buy organic food and ingredients as often as possible. Although there is controversy around cost, the more nutrient-rich the ingredients, the more satiated your body will feel with less food. This is another place to regard food as medicine. To reduce the toxic load, your body must process nutrients. And to increase the nutrient density of your food, you should have the cleanest foods you can obtain.

Beverages: Black, oolong, pu-erh, green, and herbal teas as well as homemade bone or vegetable broth

Condiments and pantry staples: Collagen peptides (grass-fed beef or marine), coconut liquid aminos, and root-based products such as cassava and tigernut flour

Dairy-free fermented foods: Kombucha, dairy-free yogurt and kefir, sauerkraut, kimchi, and vinegar

Fresh and dried herbs: Parsley, thyme, basil, tarragon, rosemary, chives, chervil, marjoram, oregano, fennel, sage, lavender, mint, cilantro, and dill

Meats: Chicken, turkey, duck, beef, pork, and lamb (organic and pasture-raised, when possible)

Non-nightshade vegetables: All vegetables except tomatoes, bell and hot peppers, eggplant, and white potatoes

Oils and fats: Avocados and avocado oil, coconut products and oil without carrageenan, extra-virgin olive oil, and clean animal fats such as pork lard, beef tallow, and duck fat

Seafood: Nearly all fish and seafood, including Alaskan salmon (never farmed), cod, mackerel, herring, trout, sardines, wild shrimp, lobster, clams, and scallops (much of our seafood is heavily burdened with toxins, so check your sources)

Foods to Moderate on the AIP

There are many nutrient-dense foods that you may be able to eat in moderation. These foods may be higher in sugar or insoluble fiber and may cause irritation or discomfort as you heal from your heightened inflammation state. So, you don't have to completely eliminate them, but you should consume them in moderation.

A diet high in sugar can increase inflammation, increase blood sugar dysregulation, disrupt normal digestion, and contribute to other issues, such as diabetes. Limiting sugar, even from sources that are still part of the elimination phase, will contribute to healing faster and feeling better.

Consume the following in moderation:

Cruciferous vegetables (one to two servings per day): Broccoli, cauliflower, kale, bok choy, and cabbage; this family of vegetables can cause gas and bloating for people with Crohn's, so small portions are key

Fresh fruit (one to two servings per day): All types with skin removed, but opt for blueberries, raspberries, and blackberries; the polyphenols they contain contribute to overall gut health

Natural sweeteners (in small amounts): Pure maple syrup, raw or Manuka honey, and coconut sugar

Unsweetened dried fruit (¼ cup per day): Take caution, as even unsweetened dried fruits can be very high in sugar

AIP SHOPPING TIPS

Shopping during the elimination phase of the AIP can feel daunting, but once you get into the rhythm of the market with your new focus, you may find it is less stressful than having to make decisions about prepared and packaged foods from dozens of brands.

Make a list and bring it with you. Stay focused and efficient.

Buy local, seasonal, and organic, where possible. Seasonal eating helps you get the most nutritional bang for your buck. It may also help inspire your meal planning.

Read food labels. For packaged foods, read labels to ensure you aren't getting grains, gums, sweeteners, and additives such as carrageenan that can cause gut irritation.

Stick to the outside of the market. All the real food is along the perimeter of the grocery store or market. Although it is impossible to avoid some aisles (such as when you need oils and spices), many of the products in the center will only make it more difficult to support your elimination phase. Having a stocked pantry and refrigerator with high-quality ingredients is less expensive than filling your cupboards with prepared and packaged foods that go to waste.

Farmers are friends. If there is a farmers' market near you, take advantage of it. Farmers always have the freshest food and often make it easier to buy organic without much fuss.

Foods to Restrict or Avoid on the AIP

The following list of foods should be removed entirely during the elimination phase of the AIP. Many of these foods are highly inflammatory or contain antinutrients, and you should consider removing them permanently to keep the impact from your Crohn's disease to a minimum and remission as a target. It is also important to avoid food additives, preservatives, and dyes. During the elimination phase, plan to get rid of most packaged and prepared food products, because your diet is going to be centered on whole, nutrient-dense foods. Avoid:

Artificial or processed meat products: bologna, cured bacon, deli meats, hot dogs, jerky, and sausages

Beverages: alcohol, soda, coffee, hot chocolate, and sweetened beverages

Dairy: milk from cows, goats, and sheep, and any food products derived from milk, such as butter, cheese, ice cream, whey protein, and yogurt

Eggs: a nutrient-dense food but a common allergen

Grains: all grains, including amaranth, barley, buckwheat, corn, kamut, millet, oats, quinoa (though technically not a grain), rice, rye, sorghum, spelt, teff, and wheat

Legumes: black beans, chickpeas, lentils, lima beans, peanuts, peas, pinto beans, and soybeans (including soy-based products like edamame, tamari, tofu, and soy milk), as well as coffee, chocolate, green beans, and snap peas

Nightshades: adobo, ancho, cayenne pepper, chili powder, curry, dried chile flakes (such as red pepper flakes), eggplants, goji berries, paprika, peppers, tomatoes, white potatoes, and most spice blends

Nuts and seeds: all nuts and seeds, including almonds, chia, flaxseed, hemp, nut butters and oils, peanuts, pumpkin, sesame, sunflower, and walnuts

Seed-derived spices: anise, annatto, black pepper, caraway, celery, coriander, cumin, dill seed, fennel, fenugreek, mustard, and nutmeg

Sweeteners: agave, artificial sweeteners (aspartame, saccharin, sucralose), barley malt, dextrose, high-fructose corn syrup, maltose, monk fruit, rice syrup, stevia, sucrose, sugar alcohols (erythritol, sorbitol, xylitol), and white sugar

Vegetable oils and trans fats: canola, corn, cottonseed, margarine, palm oils, peanut, safflower, shortening, soybean, sunflower, and all nut and seed oils

- **Fats:** avocado oil, beef tallow, coconut oil, duck fat, extra-virgin olive oil, pork fat, red palm oil
- **Fruits:** applesauce, avocados, blackberries, blueberries, olives, raspberries
- **Meat:** beef, bison, elk, goat, lamb, pork, wild boar
- **Organ meats:** bone marrow, heart, kidney, liver, oxtail, tongue, tripe
- **Poultry:** chicken, duck, quail, turkey

- **Vegetables:** acorn squash, artichoke, asparagus, beets, Brussels sprouts, butternut squash, carrots, cassava, celery, collard, cucumber, jicama, leeks, mushrooms, mustard greens, parsnips, pumpkin squash, radish, Romaine lettuce, rutabaga, scallion, seaweed, spinach, sweet potato, turnip, yam, zucchini
- **Vinegars:** apple cider, balsamic, white wine
- **Wild-caught seafood:** anchovies, bass, clams, crab, halibut, lobster, mackerel, mussels, oysters, red snapper, rockfish, sablefish, salmon, sardines, scallops, shrimp, tilapia, trout

- **Fruit:** apples with skins, bananas, cherries, dates, figs, kiwi, lemons, limes, mangos, melons, nectarines, oranges, papayas, peaches, pears, plums, strawberries, watermelons

- **Sweeteners:** coconut sugar, molasses, pure maple syrup, raw honey
- **Vegetables:** bok choy, broccoli, cabbage, cauliflower, kale (should be consumed in small amounts to avoid gas and bloating)

- **Beverages:** alcohol, coffee, hot chocolate, soda, sweetened beverages
- **Dairy:** cow, goat, and sheep milk and butter, cheese, yogurt, ice cream, whey
- **Grains:** barley, buckwheat, corn, millet, oats, quinoa, rice, rye, spelt, wheat
- **Legumes:** chickpeas, black beans, pinto beans, lima beans, lentils, peas, peanuts, soy, tofu, peas, green beans, chocolate
- **Nightshades:** bell peppers, chiles, eggplants, goji berries, tomatoes, white potatoes
- **Nuts and seeds:** almonds, cashews, chia, flaxseed, hemp, peanuts, pumpkin, sesame, sunflower, walnuts

- **Oils:** canola, corn, cottonseed, margarine, nut and seed, palm, peanut, safflower, shortening, soybean, sunflower
- **Processed meat products:** cured bacon, deli meats, hot dogs, jerky, sausages
- **Proteins:** eggs
- **Spices:** anise, annatto, black pepper, caraway, celery, coriander, cumin, dill seed, fennel, fenugreek, mustard, nutmeg
- **Sweeteners:** artificial sweeteners (aspartame, saccharin, sucralose), barley malt, dextrose, high-fructose corn syrup, maltose, monk fruit, rice syrup, stevia, sucrose, sugar alcohols (sorbitol, xylitol), white sugar

HEALTHY EATING HABITS

Eating with Crohn's is no simple matter; however, many good eating habits for people suffering from IBD are also good habits for people who don't have the disease. It is possible to have vibrant energy and digestion when living with Crohn's disease.

Evidence shows that time-restricted eating and intermittent fasting can dramatically reduce inflammation. Without putting more protocols on your plate, keep in mind that eating frequently throughout the day puts a lot of stress on your body's digestive tract. Studies, including one from 2019 published in *Cell*, show the more time you can gain between your last meal and first meal of the day, the greater the benefit. This can be even more powerful for people with Crohn's who are dealing with multifactorial issues related to digestion. Many diets recommend several small meals throughout the day, but this approach can lead to inflammation, insulin resistance, and diabetes.

Try to finish eating two hours before you go to bed and wait to eat until you start to feel hungry in the morning. Don't wait too long—to where you feel your blood sugar dropping—but if you can go twelve hours between dinner and breakfast, that is a great start to seeing some of the benefits of time-restricted eating.

Joshua has many years of experience with intermittent fasting. He usually eats his first meal at 2 or 3 p.m. and tries to be done eating at least three hours before he goes to bed. He has seen a huge benefit to how he feels as well as on inflammation levels measured by blood tests.

Stocking Your Kitchen

While you are going through the elimination phase, it is important to set yourself up for success and minimize the number of things that make it easy to stray from your goal, which is to feel better and understand which foods may be contributing to inflammation and Crohn's symptoms. The more you rid your house of items you won't eat (taking family or other household members into account, of course), the easier it will be to avoid conflicting decisions. Fill your kitchen and pantry with the nutrient-dense foods that you know contribute to your good health.

Refrigerator Items

Stocking the refrigerator with great ingredients makes it easier to make great food. Although you may choose to keep some of your proteins in the freezer, keep three to five options fresh and ready to go in the refrigerator. The following is a list of protein options and staple refrigerator items:

- Any animal-based fat product, such as pork fat, beef tallow, and duck fat

- Apples for Applesauce (page 110), blueberries, raspberries, and blackberries

- Cultured coconut yogurt, probiotics

- Fresh herbs

- Greens and non-nightshade vegetables, such as Brussels sprouts, beets, celeriac, scallions, and leeks

- Kimchi, sauerkraut, and olives

- Ripe avocados (ripen in a bag or on a shelf and then transfer to the refrigerator)

Freezer Items

Ideally, you will be eating as many fresh ingredients as possible, and if you have a nearby farmers' market, you can get away with keeping very little in the freezer. Still, it is handy to have a stash of things that are easy to pull out and use. If it is hard to find grass-fed and sustainably farmed meats and seafood locally, you may want to look into subscription services, such as ButcherBox, which give you a whole month's worth of protein. Here are some things to consider keeping on hand in the freezer:

- Hard vegetables, such as butternut squash and sweet potato, which keep well when cut and stored frozen

- Meats, such as whole chickens; beef bones for making Bone Broth (page 128); and fish

- Organic fruits and berries to enjoy out of season

Pantry Items

Stock your pantry with items used for everyday cooking. We talk later about the importance of herbs and spices for cooking and helping your body absorb nutrients from the food you eat. Your pantry should be the secret ingredients cabinet, adding flavor and nutrients to your cooking. Here are some ideas:

- Dried herbs and spices (see page 19)

- Grain-free pasta options, such as cassava

- Oils, such as avocado and extra-virgin olive oil (store solid animal-based oils in the refrigerator), as well as olives

- Vegetables that do well without refrigeration, such as cassava, winter squash, sweet potatoes, onions, shallots, and garlic

- Vinegars, such as apple cider, balsamic, and white wine

Top 10 Essentials

If you always keep these top 10 ingredients handy, you can make many of the recipes in this book, but more important, you will always have nutrient-dense food on hand for energy and healing.

1. Apples and berries

2. Aromatics such as garlic, fresh herbs, and onions

3. Bone Broth (page 128), or store-bought in a pinch

4. Coconut aminos

5. Coconut milk (no carrageenan)

6. Dark green vegetables such as kale, spinach, and chard

7. Fermented foods such as kimchi, sauerkraut, Coconut Yogurt (page 121, or store-bought)

8. Grass-fed proteins and wild fish

9. High-quality, healthy fats (fat is the most powerful metabolic engine; don't compromise and don't get too low)

10. Winter squash, cassava, and/or sweet potatoes

HERB AND SPICE CORNER

We tend to think of herbs and spices as elements that give food flavor, but they are also an important component to getting the most out of the foods we eat. The herbs and spices listed here increase nutrient absorption, are anti-inflammatory, and provide rich micronutrients that are difficult to get through other ingredients. Not all herbs and spices fit into the AIP. For example, seed-based spices may irritate or even cause additional inflammation. The herbs and spices listed here will make your food delicious:

- Basil leaves
- Bay leaves
- Chervil
- Chives
- Cilantro (leaf)
- Cinnamon
- Clove
- Dill (fresh)
- Fennel (fresh)
- Garlic
- Ginger
- Lemongrass
- Lime leaves
- Mace (a good alternative to its nut form, nutmeg)
- Marjoram
- Oregano
- Parsley
- Peppermint

- Rosemary
- Saffron
- Sage
- Salt
- Tarragon
- Thyme
- Turmeric

And here are some spices to avoid during the elimination phase:

- Allspice
- Anise seed
- Annatto seed
- Black pepper
- Caraway
- Cardamom
- Chile, dried flakes, powders, and blends containing chiles
- Coriander seed

- Cumin
- Dill seed
- Fennel seed
- Fenugreek seed
- Juniper
- Mustard seed
- Nutmeg
- Poppy seed
- Sesame seed
- Star anise
- Vanilla bean
- Wasabi and horseradish (although technically not on the "avoid" list, they are likely to irritate sensitive digestive organs, so we recommend avoiding them)

Time-Saving Tips

This book contains a mix of recipes, some easy and some more involved. Regardless of the ones you choose, there are a few tips you can always use to save time on busy days.

- Cut vegetables and store either in the refrigerator for the week or in the freezer in larger batches for later.

- Freeze fruit, such as berries, to make smoothie preparation easy.

- Use an electric pressure cooker, such as the Instant Pot brand, to make things such as Bone Broth (page 128) and slow-cooked meat.

- Plan your meals for the entire week in advance.

- Shop seasonally, ideally at a farmers' market, to have the freshest ingredients on hand.

Getting Started with Meal Planning

When making a radical change to your diet, the more prepared you are, the better. We've discussed removing items from your kitchen that don't align with the elimination phase, but there are other ways to set yourself up for success, as well.

Meal planning is a powerful tool. It helps you implement changes, making it easier to stick to your plan and gather everything you need before you get to the end of a long day. Planning your meals out a week or even two weeks at a time will ensure that when you go to the market, you have a clear sense of direction and don't get lost in the middle of the store, where all the easy and processed food items are. Having a plan is likely to save you money by reducing food waste. It also makes it easier to confirm you have a variety of nutrient-dense foods in your diet.

One of the primary factors affecting IBD and Crohn's is chronic stress, and the fewer food-related decisions you must make throughout the day, the less anxiety you are going to feel about being on a new diet. A meal plan minimizes last-minute scrambling, particularly if you have extras prepared and ready in the refrigerator.

Your meal plan can also be helpful in communicating the kinds of delicious foods you will be eating to your family and friends, and perhaps it will encourage them to eat with you to support your journey and also discover new foods.

Here, we have put together a sample two-week meal plan based on the recipes in this book. We have tried to make it easy by providing a mix of foods that are likely familiar to you as well as some more involved meals that may feel a bit more adventurous. If you are already on a high-fat diet, adjust your breakfast by removing high-carbohydrate options. Getting a significant amount of high-quality fat in the morning, with a little bit of protein, should keep your mind sharp and your body feeling good all the way until lunch. This sample plan is also designed to use foods from the previous day so you can make meals with less effort.

Here are some tips for setting up a meal plan:

- Start with what feels familiar and easy for you to prepare (and that sounds delicious!).

- Use your typical schedule to plan for more complex recipes when you have the time to enjoy making them.

- Keep your refrigerator and pantry stocked with staples that make it easy to cook when you get into the kitchen.

- Don't be too rigid; change it up with something else you've already made or that sounds good that day if you aren't in the mood for what is on the plan.

- Double recipes to have extra on hand for easy lunches and dinners.

SAMPLE 2-WEEK MEAL PLAN

WEEK 1

DAY	BREAKFAST	LUNCH	DINNER
DAY 1	½ recipe Golden Chai Latte (page 28)	Turkey Burgers with Butternut Squash Hash (page 72)	Perfect Roast Chicken with Baked Sweet Potato (page 74)
DAY 2	Butternut Squash Browns (page 37)	*Leftover* Turkey Burgers	*Leftover* Perfect Roast Chicken
DAY 3	½ recipe AIP Green Smoothie (page 30)	Nori Salmon Wraps (page 62)	Broccoli Beef Stir-Fry (page 95)
DAY 4	Leftover Skillet (page 36)	½ recipe AIP Green Smoothie	*Leftover* Broccoli Beef Stir-Fry
DAY 5	½ recipe Golden Chai Latte	*Leftover* Broccoli Beef Stir-Fry	Carnitas on Plantain Tortillas (page 98)
DAY 6	Banana Pancakes (page 33)	*Leftover* Carnitas on Plantain Tortillas	Barbecue Chicken Wings with Roasted Brussels Sprouts and Bacon (page 84)
DAY 7	*Leftover* Banana Pancakes	*Leftover* Carnitas on Plantain Tortillas	*Leftover* Barbecue Chicken Wings

WEEK 2

DAY	BREAKFAST	LUNCH	DINNER
DAY 8	½ recipe Creamy Berry and Stone Fruit Smoothie (page 29)	Sardines and Tapenade on Toast (page 106)	Chicken and Broccoli Stir-Fry with Water Chestnuts (page 77)
DAY 9	Fall Turkey B-Fast Hash (page 34)	Nori Salmon Wraps (page 62)	*Leftover* Chicken and Broccoli Stir-Fry
DAY 10	No-Oatmeal (page 31) with fruit	Avocado Toast (page 107) with fruit	Thai-Style Whitefish Curry (page 68)
DAY 11	*Leftover* No-Oatmeal with fruit	*Leftover* Thai-Style Whitefish Curry	Meatballs with Faux-Peanut Sauce and Greens (page 93)
DAY 12	Leftover Skillet (page 36)	*Leftover* Meatballs with Faux-Peanut Sauce	Buddha Bowl (page 44)
DAY 13	Cassava Waffles (page 32)	*Leftover* Buddha Bowl	Fried Chicken with Sweet Potato Waffles (page 78)
DAY 14	*Leftover* Cassava Waffles	*Leftover* Meatballs with Faux-Peanut Sauce	*Leftover* Fried Chicken with Sweet Potato Waffles

Developing Your Meal Plan

The sample two-week meal plan is just a starting point. There are many more recipes in the book that we hope you will work into your own plan throughout the elimination phase. The biggest factor for your planning is making sure you are getting a proper balance of nutrients—enough fat to keep you satiated and energetic, enough protein to ensure your body has the building blocks to make and repair cells, and enough nutrients from vegetables, herbs, and spices to ensure your body has the fiber and micronutrients to maximize absorption and repair for your gastrointestinal lining.

We tried to add enough recipes to cover most times of the year, but it can also be fun to take a trip through the market, look at what is in season, and plan your menu around what is peaking (both in flavor and nutrients). The more diversity in your foods, the more diversity in your microbiome. The fiber from the vegetables we highlight will pave the way for good bacteria to proliferate, making it easier to digest and get the most out of what you eat.

Depending on your schedule and lifestyle, you may want to plan and prepare meals in batches so you can just pull them out and reheat them. Bone Broth (page 128) is a great example of something you can make in a large batch and have on hand to make soups, which can also be made in large quantities.

If you have a sensitivity to histamine, you should minimize the number of foods you are cooking and storing in the refrigerator. In addition to histamine-producing foods, proteins in meat and vegetables start to produce histamines after they are cooked. If you are sensitive, you can minimize histamines by freezing in small batches immediately after cooking. If you find you aren't feeling well after eating leftovers that felt fine when you originally cooked them, histamines could be a culprit.

About the Recipes

The recipes in this book are intended to support you through the elimination phase of the AIP and are a good base to build from as you start to reintroduce foods. Remember, the goal is to reduce your Crohn's symptoms while having enough energy and nutrients to fuel the healing process. Nearly all foods that can be a problem for Crohn's disease have been eliminated, but that doesn't mean everything in the book will work for you. Everyone's body and gut are unique, so pay attention to how you feel, check in with your energy levels, and notice how well you are able to go about your day. Keep notes about what you liked and what you didn't to help you adjust and build the diet around your specific needs and preferences. It is important to remember that any dramatic change in your diet should be done in consultation with your health and medical team.

Tips

Many recipes include tips to make it easier to adapt them to your needs and tastes:

Ingredient tip: Provides information about specific ingredients, such as how to choose them at the peak of their freshness and when to leave them behind.

Make-ahead tip: Points out which aspects of a recipe (or the whole thing!) can be made ahead to save time.

Make it milder: Recommends substitutions that can make a recipe easier on your digestive process during flare-ups. Most recipes are already mild, but this tip points out additional adjustments.

Substitution tip: Helps you get around ingredients that may not be readily available or make dishes vegetarian or vegan.

Labels

Recipes are labeled so you can spot and mark meals that meet your needs, whether that's something quick for a weekday meal or something comforting to satisfy.

5 INGREDIENT: Recipes that use five or fewer ingredients (excluding water, salt, and oil/cooking spray).

30 MINUTES OR LESS: Recipes that can be completed in 30 minutes from start to finish—easy to cook when you don't have a lot of time.

COMFORT FOOD: Dishes that help you feel nourished emotionally and nutritionally.

ONE-POT MEAL: Cooked using only one vessel: a pot, a baking sheet, etc.

VEGETARIAN/VEGAN: Vegetarian dishes do not contain meat, and vegan dishes do not contain any animal products. In some cases, this label indicates there is a plant-based variation.

WORTH THE WAIT: Recipes that take 45 minutes or more from start to finish but are so good, you won't mind the extra effort.

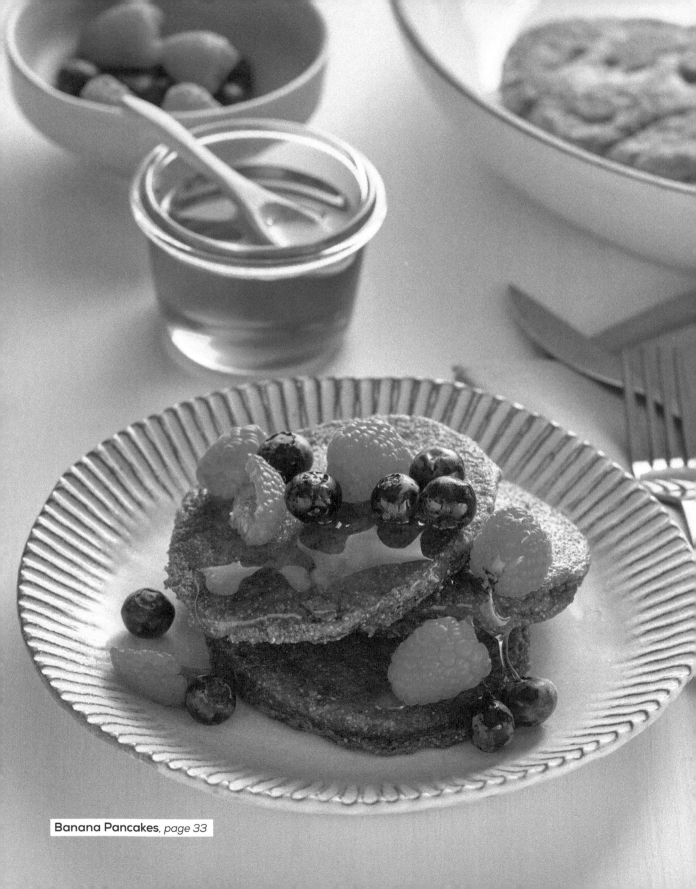

Banana Pancakes, *page 33*

CHAPTER 3

BREAKFAST AND SMOOTHIES

GOLDEN CHAI LATTE

30 MINUTES OR LESS **VEGAN OPTION**

Serves 2 / **Prep time:** 10 minutes

Made with healthy fat and spices, this latte is a great way to get your morning started. The spices used are all powerful immune boosters, and cinnamon and clove help regulate blood sugar. Turmeric is best absorbed by the body when combined with fat, making this latte a perfect way to get the powerful anti-inflammatory into your diet.

1 tablespoon black tea (such as Assam)

½ teaspoon ground ginger or ½-inch piece fresh ginger

16 ounces boiling water

8 ounces coconut milk (no gums or carrageenan)

2 scoops/servings grass-fed/finished collagen peptides (optional, see Resources, page 140)

1 teaspoon honey or another AIP-approved sweetener (optional)

1 teaspoon ground turmeric

½ teaspoon ground cinnamon

⅛ teaspoon ground cloves

1. Add the black tea and ginger to the boiling water and steep for 3 minutes off the heat.

2. Strain the tea and transfer to a blender. Add the coconut milk, collagen (if using), honey (if using), turmeric, cinnamon, and cloves.

3. Blend for at least 30 seconds, then serve.

INGREDIENT TIP: MCT oil derived from coconuts could be added to boost ketone production but should be consumed in smaller quantities to start if you are not used to it. Kia recommends to stop using MCT by 3 p.m. because it's energizing and can interrupt sleep if consumed late in the day. Omit the tea, and this golden milk could improve your sleep thanks to the nourishing and gut-soothing ingredients.

MAKE-AHEAD TIP: If using ground ginger, make a spice blend by scaling up the cloves, cinnamon, and ginger and mix well. Use a slightly heaping teaspoon of the blend when you make your latte.

PER SERVING: Calories: 212; Total fat: 21g; Carbohydrates: 8g; Fiber: 2g; Protein: 2g; Sodium: 13mg

CREAMY BERRY AND STONE FRUIT SMOOTHIE

30 MINUTES OR LESS | ONE-POT MEAL | VEGAN OPTION

Serves 2 / Prep time: 5 minutes

This delicious berry smoothie packs a serious antioxidant punch. Blueberries and raspberries have been shown to have a positive impact on the gut microbiome, and, when combined with coconut yogurt, they make a perfectly yummy way to build gut health.

Juice of ½ lemon

½ Granny Smith apple, cored, skin on

½ teaspoon maqui berry powder (optional)

2 cups Coconut Yogurt (page 121, or store-bought)

1 cup fresh or frozen nectarine, peach, or apricot, stone and skin removed

½ cup frozen blueberries

½ cup frozen raspberries or blackberries

2 scoops/servings grass-fed/finished collagen peptides (optional, see Resources, page 140)

½ cup ice (optional, if using fresh fruit)

1. In a blender, combine the lemon juice, apple, berry powder (if using), coconut yogurt, nectarine, blueberries, raspberries, and collagen (if using). If using fresh fruit, add the ice. Blend until smooth.

2. Add cold water, as needed, to reach the desired consistency.

INGREDIENT TIP: If using store-bought unsweetened coconut yogurt, be sure there is no maltodextrin derived from corn or carrageenan. Choose organic berries and fruit.

MAKE-AHEAD TIP: Smoothies are best when fresh because the nutrients start to break down the moment everything gets blended. You can make this the night before and pluck it out of the refrigerator in the morning for an on-the-go breakfast, but don't keep smoothies for more than a day.

PER SERVING: Calories: 491; Total fat: 36g; Carbohydrates: 44g; Fiber: 9g; Protein: 7g; Sodium: 41mg

AIP GREEN SMOOTHIE

30 MINUTES OR LESS ONE-POT MEAL VEGAN OPTION

Serves 2 / **Prep time:** 5 minutes

This smoothie provides a tremendous number of micronutrients without any cooking. Because you are consuming raw ingredients, it is even more important to make sure that you are buying the freshest available and choosing organic.

6 parsley sprigs

4 large kale or rainbow chard leaves, stemmed, or 2 cups spinach

2 scoops/servings grass-fed/finished collagen peptides (optional, see Resources, page 140)

Juice of ½ lemon

½ ripe avocado

½ Granny Smith apple, cored, skin on

½ cup frozen blueberries

2 teaspoons moringa powder (optional)

1 cup ice

1. In a blender, combine the parsley, kale, collagen (if using), lemon juice, avocado, apple, blueberries, and moringa (if using). Add the ice and blend until smooth.

2. Add cold water, as needed, to reach the desired consistency.

INGREDIENT TIP: If you have access to a juice shop that has fresh-pressed ginger and turmeric juice, add 1 tablespoon of one or both to boost the anti-inflammatory, gut-healing powers of this smoothie. Moringa powder is made from a super nutrient- and antioxidant-rich leaf, originating in Africa, that has been shown to reduce inflammation and help control blood sugars.

MAKE-AHEAD TIP: Smoothies are best when fresh, as the nutrients start to break down the moment everything gets blended. You can make one the night before and pluck it out of the refrigerator in morning for an on-the-go breakfast, but don't keep smoothies for more than a day.

PER SERVING: Calories: 121; Total fat: 6g; Carbohydrates: 18g; Fiber: 6g; Protein: 2g; Sodium: 16mg

NO-OATMEAL

5 INGREDIENT   30 MINUTES OR LESS   COMFORT FOOD   VEGAN OPTION

Serves 2 / **Prep time:** 5 minutes / **Cook time:** 3 minutes

Oatmeal is one of the great morning comfort foods. This grain-free version will give you all the same feels but will feed your gut and keep inflammation down. Tigernuts are not actually nuts but are tubers about the size of a chickpea, originally cultivated in Egypt. Tigernuts are high in insoluble fiber and resistant starch, making them a great prebiotic food.

½ cup water

½ cup coconut flakes

½ cup tigernut flour

2 scoops/servings grass-fed/finished collagen peptides (optional, see Resources, page 140)

1 teaspoon honey or other AIP-approved sweetener

1 apple, chopped and cooked until soft with cinnamon (optional)

½ cup berries (optional)

½ cup Coconut Yogurt (page 121; optional)

¼ teaspoon ground cinnamon (optional)

1. In a medium saucepan, bring the water to a boil over medium-high heat.

2. Combine the coconut and tigernut flour in a food processor or blender and pulse until the coconut is coarse, like grains of rice. Transfer to the boiling water.

3. Add the collagen (if using) and honey. Reduce the heat to low and cook for 3 minutes or until thickened. Add more water, as necessary, to reach the desired consistency.

4. Divide between two bowls and top with the apple, berries, coconut yogurt, and cinnamon (if using). Serve warm.

INGREDIENT TIP: Boost the nutrient and anti-inflammatory powers by adding 2 teaspoons of moringa powder and/or ½ teaspoon of ground turmeric. Due to the high fiber content, start out eating smaller amounts of no-oatmeal to avoid producing gas.

SUBSTITUTION TIP: For a richer no-oatmeal, replace the water with 8 ounces of coconut milk.

PER SERVING: Calories: 273; Total fat: 20g; Carbohydrates: 22g; Fiber: 6g; Protein: 2g; Sodium: 8mg

CASSAVA WAFFLES

30 MINUTES OR LESS   COMFORT FOOD   VEGAN OPTION

Makes 3 large waffles / **Prep time:** 10 minutes / **Cook time:** 15 minutes

Because of its high starch content, cassava flour makes a great waffle that crisps up on the outside but remains soft on the inside. These waffles have no grains, eggs, or dairy but will leave you completely satisfied.

1 cup whole cassava flour

2 tablespoons tigernut flour or green banana flour

1 scoop/serving grass-fed/finished collagen peptides (optional, see Resources, page 140)

1 teaspoon baking powder

¼ teaspoon baking soda

¼ teaspoon sea salt

1 cup coconut milk (no gums or carrageenan)

2 tablespoons avocado oil or melted coconut oil

1. Preheat a waffle maker.

2. In a large bowl, whisk together the cassava flour, tigernut flour, collagen (if using), baking powder, baking soda, and salt. In a small bowl, whisk together the coconut milk and oil until well blended, then add to the flour mixture and blend until smooth. The batter should be thick but pourable. If needed, thin it with some water.

3. Pour one-third of the batter onto the center of the waffle maker until three-fourths of the surface is covered. Close the waffle maker and cook for 3 minutes. Remove the waffle and set aside. Repeat this process with the remaining batter, then serve warm.

INGREDIENT TIP: Add moringa powder to up the nutrients. Top with smoothie ingredients, such as coconut yogurt, fresh berries, or peeled and sliced stone fruit. For a savory approach, add rendered and chopped uncured bacon to the batter or serve with breakfast sausage.

MAKE-AHEAD TIP: Waffles can be made ahead and kept in the freezer. Toast them in a toaster for a quick breakfast.

PER WAFFLE: Calories: 379; Total fat: 24g; Carbohydrates: 42g; Fiber: 4g; Protein: 2g; Sodium: 474mg

BANANA PANCAKES

30 MINUTES OR LESS COMFORT FOOD **VEGAN OPTION**
Makes 6 to 10 pancakes / **Prep time:** 5 minutes / **Cook time:** 25 minutes

Berries and sliced fruit are always a good option for toppings, but pancakes aren't quite the same without a little maple syrup. Don't go overboard; too much sugar can easily upset the balance of good bacteria building in the gut.

2 tablespoons avocado oil or melted coconut oil, plus more for greasing

½ cup Coconut Yogurt (page 121, or store-bought)

1 banana, just ripe, or ripe plantain

1 cup whole cassava flour

2 tablespoons green banana flour

2 scoops/servings grass-fed/finished collagen peptides (optional, see Resources, page 140)

½ teaspoon baking powder

½ teaspoon baking soda

¼ teaspoon sea salt

1. Lightly grease a griddle or cast-iron pan with oil, then place over medium heat.

2. In a blender, combine the coconut yogurt, oil, and banana and puree until smooth. Add the cassava and banana flours, collagen (if using), baking powder, baking soda, and salt and blend until smooth. The batter should be thick but pourable. If needed, thin it with some water.

3. Test the heat of the griddle with a few drops of water. It should pop and sizzle in little beads. Pour ½ cup of batter onto the griddle. It should spread out to get at least 30 percent bigger. If the batter remains in a lump, mix a bit of water into the rest of the batter.

4. Cook for 2 minutes or until the edges become dull (no longer wet and glossy) and bubbles start to form but not pop. Flip and continue cooking for 1 to 2 minutes, until the center is firm.

5. Transfer the pancake to a plate, then repeat this process with the remaining batter. Serve warm.

MAKE-AHEAD TIP: Pancakes can be made ahead and kept in the freezer. Reheat in an oven or microwave for a quick breakfast.

PER PANCAKE (1 OF 6): Calories: 171; Total fat: 8g; Carbohydrates: 27g; Fiber: 2g; Protein: 1g; Sodium: 248mg

FALL TURKEY B-FAST HASH

30 MINUTES OR LESS **ONE-POT MEAL**

Serves 1 / **Prep time:** 5 minutes / **Cook time:** 25 minutes

Turkey has a different amino acid profile than other meat and poultry, as it is higher in gut-healthy tryptophan and the cell-building powerhouses lysine and arginine, which are vital for protein synthesis.

1 tablespoon solid fat, such as coconut oil or pork fat, divided

4 ounces ground or leftover turkey

1 fennel bulb, halved and cut into rings

½ small onion, cut into half-moons

Sea salt

1 cup cubed butternut squash or sweet potato

¼ cup water

1 rosemary sprig

1 tablespoon chopped fresh parsley

½ teaspoon ground sage, or 3 or 4 sage leaves, thinly sliced

1. In a large skillet over medium heat, warm ½ tablespoon of oil.

2. If using ground turkey, add it to the skillet and cook for about 15 minutes, breaking it up with a wooden spoon, until lightly browned. Transfer to a plate and set aside.

3. Add the remaining ½ tablespoon of oil, the fennel, the onion, and a pinch of salt. Cook for about 3 minutes, until the onion is translucent and starting to brown. Add the squash, mixing to make sure it is in a single layer and not too crowded in the pan. Cook for 1 minute, then stir. You may need to scrape the squash from the bottom of the pan.

4. Add the water, scraping up all the browned bits. Add the rosemary, parsley, and sage, cover, and reduce the heat to low. Steam for about 5 minutes, until the squash is tender.

5. Add the reserved turkey. Taste and add salt as needed. Cook, stirring, for 1 minute, then serve.

MAKE-AHEAD TIP: Precook cubes of butternut squash or sweet potato and keep small amounts in the refrigerator or larger amounts in the freezer.

PER SERVING: Calories: 498; Total fat: 29g; Carbohydrates: 43g; Fiber: 15g; Protein: 24g; Sodium: 195mg

SWEET POTATO, AVOCADO, AND SEAWEED BOWL

COMFORT FOOD   VEGAN OPTION

Serves 2 / **Prep time:** 10 minutes / **Cook time:** 30 minutes

Keep the flavors from the ginger and garlic light, and let the umami from the vinaigrette and seaweed drive the flavor in this nutrient-packed dish.

1 cup cubed peeled sweet potato

2 tablespoons avocado oil, divided

½ teaspoon coarse salt, divided

4 ounces ground pork, chicken, or turkey

1 garlic clove, minced

½ teaspoon minced fresh ginger

1 scallion, green part only, cut into thin rounds

2 teaspoons coconut aminos

2 tablespoons dulse or wakame flakes, soaked in warm water for 5 minutes

½ avocado, cut into ¼-inch-thick slices

. . . .

PER SERVING: Calories: 460; Total fat: 31g; Carbohydrates: 33g; Fiber: 8g; Protein: 14g; Sodium: 729mg

1. Place a rimmed baking sheet in the oven and preheat it to 375°F.

2. In a medium bowl, toss together the sweet potato, 1 tablespoon of oil, and ¼ teaspoon of salt. Open the oven and spread the sweet potato on the hot baking sheet. Roast for about 30 minutes, until tender and browning.

3. Meanwhile, in the same bowl, mix together the pork, garlic, ginger, and the remaining ¼ teaspoon of salt until well combined. Form into ½-inch balls.

4. Heat ½ teaspoon of oil in a large skillet over medium heat. When hot, add the meatballs and cook for 3 to 5 minutes, until browned on all sides and cooked through. Remove and set aside.

5. Pour the remaining 2½ teaspoons of oil into a small bowl and whisk in the scallion and coconut aminos.

6. Divide the roasted sweet potatoes between two bowls. Top with the meatballs followed by the seaweed and avocado, then pour the vinaigrette over the top. Serve.

INGREDIENT TIP: Use nori, a seaweed used in sushi and seaweed snack packs, if it is easier to find than dulse.

SUBSTITUTION TIP: To make this vegan, use finely chopped portobello mushrooms instead of ground meat.

LEFTOVER SKILLET

5 INGREDIENT   30 MINUTES OR LESS   ONE-POT MEAL   VEGAN OPTION
Serves 1 / **Prep time:** 5 minutes / **Cook time:** 15 minutes

The leftover skillet can be deftly deployed as a midweek savior when you are starting to run out of ideas, but it is equally useful to take stock of the refrigerator on Sunday morning and free up some space for the following week. Let what you made for the week inspire your breakfast, mix-and-match vegetables and proteins, and then embellish with flavors you're in the mood for.

2 uncured/nitrate-free bacon slices (optional)

1 tablespoon avocado or coconut oil (optional)

½ cup leftover starchy vegetables, such as squash, sweet potato, plantains, or cassava

½ cup soft vegetables, such as cauliflower, collards or kale, beets, Brussels sprouts, or bok choy

4 ounces leftover protein, such as shredded chicken, pulled pork, beef, duck, fish, or portobello mushrooms

Sea salt

2 tablespoons refrigerator staples, such as kimchi or sauerkraut, pesto, or guacamole

Chopped fresh herbs of choice, for garnish (optional)

1. In a medium skillet over medium heat, cook the bacon (if using) for about 7 minutes, flipping as needed, until crisp. Transfer to a plate and reserve the fat in the pan. If not using bacon, pour the avocado or coconut oil into the skillet.

2. Add the starchy vegetables and cook over medium heat for 2 to 3 minutes. Add the soft vegetables and protein and cook for 2 to 3 minutes. Taste and add salt as needed.

3. Transfer to a plate, top with the refrigerator staple, garnish with herbs (if using), and serve.

Nutritional content will vary based on ingredients used.

BUTTERNUT SQUASH BROWNS

5 INGREDIENT **30 MINUTES OR LESS** **VEGAN OPTION**

Serves 1 / Prep time: 5 minutes / **Cook time:** 20 minutes

Butternut squash makes a great breakfast brown with fewer calories, carbohydrates, and sugar than sweet potato. Embellish this dish with a leftover protein, such as Barbecue Jackfruit (page 46), Bolognese sauce (page 90), or Cuban-Style Picadillo (page 100).

2 uncured/nitrate-free bacon slices, cut into ½-inch wide strips (optional; see tip)

1 cup shredded butternut squash

1 teaspoon tapioca starch

1 teaspoon chopped fresh parsley

½ teaspoon chopped fresh sage

¼ teaspoon coarse salt

1. In a medium skillet over medium heat, cook the bacon (if using) for about 7 minutes, flipping as needed, until crisp. Transfer to a plate. Keep half of the fat in the pan and set the remaining half aside.

2. Meanwhile, in a medium bowl, toss together the squash, tapioca starch, parsley, sage, and salt.

3. Return the pan with the bacon fat to the heat and make sure it is sizzling hot. Arrange the seasoned squash in the center of the pan, like a pancake.

4. Cook for 5 minutes, until the bottom of the squash is browned. Use a spatula to remove the squash from the pan. Add the reserved fat, swirling to coat the pan, then return the squash, uncooked-side down, to the pan. Cook for another 5 minutes, until tender. If the squash needs more time after 5 minutes, reduce the temperature to low, cover, and let cook until the squash is tender. Serve.

SUBSTITUTION TIP: To make a vegan version, omit the bacon and swap in ½ cup of sliced mushrooms and 1 teaspoon of coconut oil and cook until the water releases and the mushrooms are soft.

PER SERVING: Calories: 167; Total fat: 5g; Carbohydrates: 25g; Fiber: 7g; Protein: 8g; Sodium: 441mg

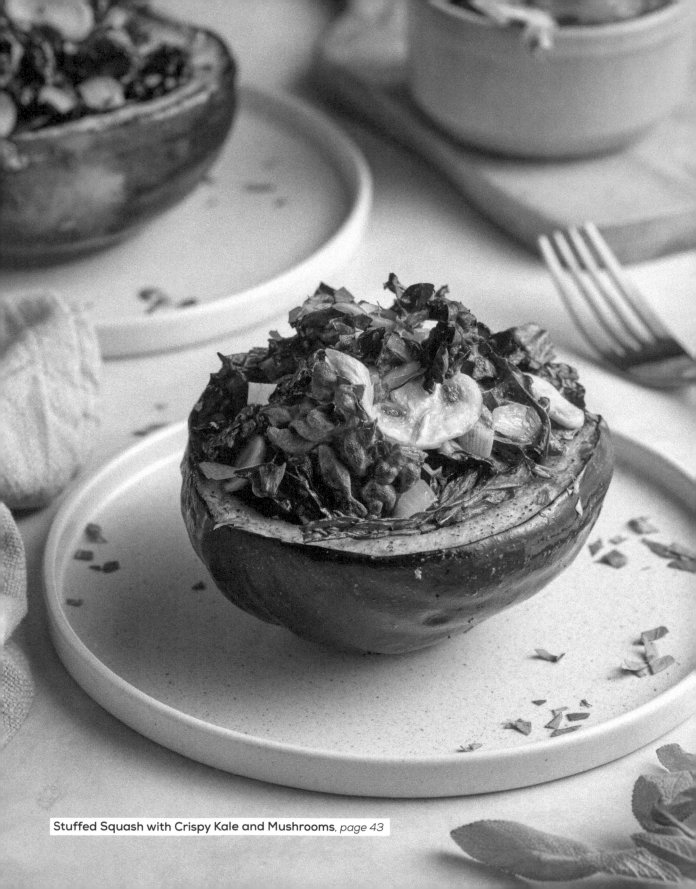

Stuffed Squash with Crispy Kale and Mushrooms, *page 43*

CHAPTER 4

VEGETARIAN AND VEGAN MAINS

VEGETABLE CURRY

30 MINUTES OR LESS **VEGAN**

Serves 2 / **Prep time:** 10 minutes / **Cook time:** 20 minutes

Curry is a perfect nutrient delivery system—warm, rich, and delicious. The spices provide flavor and powerful anti-inflammatory properties that, when combined, are more easily absorbed by the body.

3 tablespoons coconut oil, divided

2 garlic cloves, chopped

1 carrot, thinly sliced on the bias

½ onion, sliced lengthwise

½-inch piece fresh ginger, minced or grated

Sea salt

1 teaspoon ground turmeric

½ teaspoon ground cinnamon

⅛ teaspoon ground cloves

8 ounces coconut milk (no gums or carrageenan)

2 cups cauliflower or cassava rice

½ pound cremini mushrooms, stemmed

2 tablespoons coconut aminos

1 tablespoon chopped fresh cilantro

Juice of ½ lime

1 scallion, green part only, cut into rounds

1. In a large skillet over medium-high heat, warm 1 tablespoon of oil. Add the garlic, carrot, onion, ginger, and a pinch of salt. Cook, mixing frequently, for about 2 minutes, until the onion is translucent and starting to brown.

2. Clear a spot in the center of the skillet and add the turmeric, cinnamon, and cloves. When fragrant, stir in the coconut milk and bring to a simmer.

3. Meanwhile, in a medium pan over medium heat, warm the cauliflower rice and 1 tablespoon of oil. Transfer to a serving bowl.

4. In a separate medium pan over high heat, warm the remaining 1 tablespoon of oil. Add the mushrooms and cook for 1 minute. Flip and continue cooking for 2 to 3 minutes, until they start to soften and reduce. Transfer to the curry sauce, mixing to incorporate. Add the coconut aminos, cilantro, and lime juice. Taste and add salt as needed.

5. Top the cauliflower rice with the curry. Garnish with the scallion, then serve.

SUBSTITUTION TIP: Replace the rice with 1 cup of cubed sweet potato, roasted or reheated in a pan with 1 tablespoon of oil.

PER SERVING: Calories: 499; Total fat: 42g; Carbohydrates: 27g; Fiber: 7g; Protein: 9g; Sodium: 339mg

ROASTED BUTTERNUT SQUASH SOUP

VEGAN

Makes 8 servings / **Prep time:** 10 minutes / **Cook time:** 30 minutes

Butternut squash soup is a perfect dish to keep in quart-size mason jars in the refrigerator. Eat as a side dish with another meal or big salad, or reheat it in a big bowl for a satisfying lunch.

1 butternut squash, halved and seeded

1 leek, trimmed

1 tablespoon avocado or coconut oil

1 teaspoon sea salt

3 to 4 cups no-bone broth (see Substitution tip, page 128)

2 garlic cloves, chopped

1-inch piece fresh ginger, smashed and minced, or ½ teaspoon ground ginger

1 teaspoon ground turmeric (optional)

½ cup coconut milk (no gums or carrageenan)

2 tablespoons coconut cream from can of coconut milk

1. Preheat the oven to 375°F.

2. Brush the squash halves and leek with the oil and season with the salt. Transfer to a rimmed baking sheet and roast for about 30 minutes, until browned and soft. Remove from the oven and let cool.

3. Meanwhile, in a soup pot over medium-high heat, bring the broth to a simmer. Reserve 1 cup and set aside.

4. Spoon the roasted squash from its skin into a blender. Coarsely chop the leek and add it to the blender with the garlic, ginger, and turmeric (if using). Add the coconut milk and puree until smooth. Slowly add hot broth from the pot, fully incorporating it. When your blender reaches its capacity for hot liquid, split the remaining broth into two pots and divide the puree equally between both pots. Return each to the blender to puree before combining both batches in a single soup pot.

5. Taste and add salt as needed. If too thick, add the reserved 1 cup of heated broth.

6. Serve the coconut cream on top or swirled into the soup.

PER SERVING: Calories: 98; Total fat: 5g; Carbohydrates: 14g; Fiber: 4g; Protein: 1g; Sodium: 351mg

RATATOUILLE

ONE-POT MEAL   VEGAN   WORTH THE WAIT

Serves 4 / **Prep time:** 15 minutes / **Cook time:** 40 minutes

Ratatouille is summer's bounty cooked in a single pot until the flavors meld into something greater than its parts. Feel free to let what's in season inspire you—just make sure you avoid those nightshades! This recipe keeps well in the refrigerator, so double it up for leftovers.

¼ cup extra-virgin olive oil

2 or 3 golden beets (about ½ pound), peeled and cut into ½-inch dice

3 carrots (about ½ pound), peeled and cut into ½-inch dice

4 garlic cloves, minced

1 large red onion, cut into ½-inch dice

2 cups No-Mato Sauce (page 122)

1 or 2 yellow summer squash, cut into ½-inch dice

1 or 2 zucchini, cut into ½-inch dice

1 tablespoon dried oregano

1 teaspoon dried thyme

1 bay leaf

1 teaspoon sea salt

Fresh basil, for garnish (optional)

1. Preheat the oven to 375°F.

2. In a large ovenproof saucepan over medium-low heat, warm the oil. Add the beets and carrots, cover, and cook for 10 minutes. Add the garlic and onion and sauté for 1 minute. Add the no-mato sauce to the pan along with the squash, zucchini, oregano, thyme, bay leaf, and salt, mixing well.

3. Put the saucepan in the oven to bake for 30 minutes or until the vegetables are tender.

4. Remove from the oven, discard the bay leaf, and garnish with the basil (if using). Serve.

MAKE-AHEAD TIP: Make the no-mato sauce ahead of time. It's a good idea to have a jar in the refrigerator at all times.

PER SERVING: Calories: 393; Total fat: 29g; Carbohydrates: 32g; Fiber: 7g; Protein: 6g; Sodium: 1,280mg

STUFFED SQUASH WITH CRISPY KALE AND MUSHROOMS

VEGAN   WORTH THE WAIT

Serves 2 / **Prep time:** 15 minutes / **Cook time:** 55 minutes

This dish capitalizes on the ultimate flavors of fall with sage and mace. The mushrooms and kale provide a nutrient boost as well as a nice textural contrast.

1 acorn squash

1 tablespoon extra-virgin olive oil, divided, plus more for brushing the squash

Sea salt

1 pinch mace

2 shallots, chopped

¼ cup chopped fresh sage

3 garlic cloves, minced

1 cup mushrooms, cleaned and sliced

2 cups chopped lacinato or curly kale leaves

1 tablespoon chopped fresh parsley

. . . .

PER SERVING: Calories: 210; Total fat: 7g; Carbohydrates: 36g; Fiber: 7g; Protein: 6g; Sodium: 42mg

1. Preheat the oven to 400°F.

2. Halve the acorn squash lengthwise. Scoop out and discard the seeds. Brush the acorn squash halves with oil and sprinkle with salt and the mace.

3. Put the squash on a rimmed baking sheet, cut-side up, and roast for 30 to 40 minutes, until very tender when pierced with a knife.

4. Meanwhile, in a medium skillet over medium heat, warm 2 teaspoons of oil. Add the shallots with a pinch of salt and cook for 2 to 3 minutes, until translucent. Add the sage and garlic and cook for 1 minute. Add the mushrooms and cook until the mushrooms release their liquid and it has mostly evaporated from the pan, 2 to 3 minutes.

5. In a medium bowl, toss the kale with the remaining 1 teaspoon of oil and a pinch of salt to coat. Add the mushroom mixture and toss to combine.

6. When the squash is ready, remove the baking sheet from the oven but keep the heat on. If you have a convection setting on the oven, turn it to 400°F.

7. Fill the squash halves with the kale-mushroom stuffing. Return the baking sheet to the oven and roast for 10 to 15 minutes, until the squash is browned and the kale is crisp. Sprinkle with the parsley and serve.

BUDDHA BOWL

30 MINUTES OR LESS **COMFORT FOOD** **VEGAN**

Serves 2 / **Prep time:** 15 minutes / **Cook time:** 15 minutes

The Buddha bowl has become a food blog sensation. My version is based on a dish from the now-closed Dragonfly Cafe and Gardens in Ashland, Oregon. Buddha bowls are about maximizing the amount of nutrients in a fresh and vibrant bowl of food.

2 to 3 cups no-bone broth (see Substitution tip, page 128)

2 garlic cloves, chopped

1 lemongrass stalk, smashed and cut into 2-inch lengths

1-inch piece fresh ginger, smashed

½ cup coconut milk (no gums or carrageenan)

2 tablespoons coconut aminos

½ teaspoon sea salt, plus more as needed

Vegetable-based noodles, such as spaghetti squash or spiralized zucchini

1 tablespoon avocado or coconut oil

2 celery stalks, thinly sliced on the bias

1. In a medium saucepan over medium-high heat, combine the broth, garlic, lemongrass, ginger, coconut milk, coconut aminos, and ½ teaspoon of salt and bring to a simmer. Adjust the heat as needed to maintain a simmer.

2. Meanwhile, bring a separate medium saucepan of water to a boil over medium-high heat. Add the noodles and cook for about 1 minute, until tender. Drain and reserve.

3. Heat the oil in a wok over high heat or in a large skillet over medium-high heat. Add the celery, carrot, onion, and a pinch of salt and cook, stirring frequently, for about 3 minutes, until the onion is translucent and starting to brown. Transfer to a bowl.

4. Add the seasonal vegetables, mushrooms, and a pinch of salt to the wok and cook until tender. Return the onion mixture to the wok and reheat for 1 minute. Remove from the heat.

1 carrot, thinly sliced on the bias

½ onion, sliced lengthwise

½ cup seasonal vegetables, cut into 2-inch pieces

½ cup sliced fresh mushrooms

1 tablespoon cilantro pesto (see Substitution tip, page 120)

1 scallion, green part only, cut into rounds

5. Assemble two bowls by dividing the noodles evenly between them. Top each with half of the vegetable mix.

6. Taste the broth and add salt as needed. Strain the broth and pour half of the liquid over each bowl. Top with a dollop of cilantro pesto and the scallion. Serve.

INGREDIENT TIP: Make a quick version by having vegetables prepped and precooked or by using reheated leftover vegetables with the broth poured over.

SUBSTITUTION TIP: Replace the noodles with cauliflower or cassava rice and reduce the amount of broth to make it more of a sauce to pour around the ingredients. Instead of fresh mushrooms, use dried mushrooms reconstituted in hot water for 5 minutes.

PER SERVING: Calories: 250; Total fat: 24g; Carbohydrates: 18g; Fiber: 4g; Protein: 5g; Sodium: 1,367mg

BARBECUE JACKFRUIT WITH CELERIAC SLAW

30 MINUTES OR LESS   **VEGETARIAN**

Serves 2 / **Prep time:** 20 minutes / **Cook time:** 10 minutes

Jackfruit is surprisingly satisfying as a meat replacement, especially in this barbecue-style dish. Serve over a baked sweet potato or cauliflower rice with slaw on the side.

FOR THE CELERIAC SLAW

½ celeriac, cleaned and shredded

6 Brussels sprouts, washed, trimmed, and very thinly sliced

1 carrot, peeled and shredded

1 scallion, cut into 2-inch lengths, then lengthwise into very thin strips

1 tablespoon chopped fresh cilantro

1 tablespoon freshly squeezed lemon juice

3 tablespoons apple cider vinegar

2 tablespoons extra-virgin olive oil

½ teaspoon honey or maple syrup

¼ teaspoon sea salt

⅛ teaspoon horseradish or wasabi powder (optional)

TO MAKE THE CELERIAC SLAW

1. In a large bowl, combine the celeriac, Brussels sprouts, carrot, scallion, and cilantro. Add the lemon juice and mix to combine.

2. In a small bowl, whisk together the vinegar, oil, honey, salt, and horseradish (if using). Add the mixture to the slaw and stir well. Taste and adjust the seasoning as needed. Set aside.

TO MAKE THE BARBECUE JACKFRUIT

3. In a medium saucepan over medium heat, bring the no-mato sauce to a simmer. Add the garlic, onion, honey, molasses, oregano, and ¼ teaspoon of salt. Cook for 3 minutes. Taste and add the remaining ¼ teaspoon of salt if needed.

FOR THE JACKFRUIT

1 cup No-Mato Sauce
(page 122)

1 garlic clove, minced

½ onion, minced

¼ cup honey or maple syrup

1 tablespoon blackstrap
molasses

1 teaspoon dried oregano

½ teaspoon smoked salt,
divided

1 large can jackfruit in water
or ½ pound frozen plain
jackfruit, thawed

4. Add the jackfruit and cook for about 7 minutes, until the jackfruit is heated through and the sauce is thick. Stir as needed to coat the jackfruit. Serve.

INGREDIENT TIP: Jackfruit can be found fresh, but it's hard to work with. I recommend canned or frozen options.

MAKE IT MILDER: If you are having a flare-up, omit the horseradish.

PER SERVING: Calories: 604; Total fat: 28g; Carbohydrates: 85g; Fiber: 15g; Protein: 7g; Sodium: 1,643mg

WILTED KALE SALAD WITH APPLE

30 MINUTES OR LESS **ONE-POT MEAL** **VEGETARIAN**
Serves 2 / **Prep time:** 10 minutes / **Cook time:** 5 minutes

Kale is one of the most nutrient-dense foods available, but it can be difficult to digest. Wilting the kale in a bit of broth makes it easier to digest and to absorb its nutrients. Kale is rich in vitamins A, C, and K; calcium; and folate; and it has nearly 3 grams of protein per cup.

1 tablespoon organic vinegar

1 tablespoon extra-virgin olive oil

½ teaspoon honey or maple syrup

½ teaspoon sea salt, plus a pinch

¼ cup no-bone broth (see Substitution tip, page 128)

1 to 2 garlic cloves, minced

½ pound kale, stemmed and leaves halved

2 small apples, cored, peeled, and cut into matchsticks

½ small jicama, peeled and cut into matchsticks

2 tablespoons currants or dried cranberries

1. In a small bowl, whisk together the vinegar, oil, honey, and a pinch of salt.

2. In a large saucepan over medium heat, combine the broth, garlic, and half of the vinaigrette. Add the kale and the remaining ½ teaspoon of salt. Stir to coat the leaves. Cover and steam for 2 to 3 minutes or until wilted. Divide between two large salad bowls or plates.

3. Toss the apples and jicama with the remaining vinaigrette. Top each salad with half of the apple mixture and currants. Serve.

INGREDIENT TIP: Make the salad even easier by using packaged baby kale that doesn't have the woody stems. Add seasonal vegetables that complement the flavors, such as asparagus, artichoke hearts, or ripe avocado.

PER SERVING: Calories: 233; Total fat: 9g; Carbohydrates: 39g; Fiber: 11g; Protein: 5g; Sodium: 669mg

CASSAVA FRIED RICE

30 MINUTES OR LESS **VEGAN**

Serves 2 / **Prep time:** 15 minutes / **Cook time:** 15 minutes

This dish is inspired by kappa puttu, an Indian shredded cassava and coconut cake. We don't want the rice to stick to itself the way it does in the cake, so we've omitted the coconut and use the technique of grating and steaming cassava.

2 cups freshly grated cassava root

2 tablespoons avocado or coconut oil, divided

2 celery stalks, finely diced

2 garlic cloves, minced

1 carrot, finely diced

½ onion, finely diced

½ cup asparagus, cut into 1-inch pieces

½ cup summer squash, finely diced

½ cup sliced fresh mushrooms

1 teaspoon minced fresh ginger

2 tablespoons coconut aminos

¼ teaspoon sea salt

1 scallion, green part only, cut into rounds

1. In a large pot over medium-high heat, bring 2 inches of water to a simmer. Place a fine mesh basket or strainer on top of the pot. Adjust the heat as needed to maintain the simmer.

2. Put the cassava in the basket, cover, and steam for 10 minutes. Remove and let cool.

3. Meanwhile, heat a wok or large skillet over high heat. Add 1 tablespoon of oil and swirl it around. Add the celery, garlic, carrot, onion, asparagus, squash, mushrooms, and ginger, and cook, stirring frequently, for about 3 minutes or until the carrots are tender. Remove from the heat and transfer everything to a large bowl.

4. Heat the remaining 1 tablespoon of oil in the wok. Add the cassava and stir-fry for 30 seconds before returning the veggie mixture to the wok. Add the coconut aminos and salt and mix.

5. Taste and add more salt or coconut aminos as needed. Serve in a bowl topped with the scallion.

SUBSTITUTION TIP: Replace the cassava with cauliflower rice. Cauliflower rice can be used anywhere you use cassava rice.

PER SERVING: Calories: 521; Total fat: 15g; Carbohydrates: 93g; Fiber: 7g; Protein: 6g; Sodium: 652mg

MOFONGO WITH VEGETABLE STEW

30 MINUTES OR LESS **VEGAN**

Serves 4 / **Prep time:** 10 minutes / **Cook time:** 20 minutes

Mofongo is a dish of mashed plantains most often associated with Puerto Rico and the Dominican Republic, with roots in Africa. Plantains are tremendously beneficial for gut health; when unripe (green), they're a good source of resistant starch that helps pave the way for good bacteria to grow.

FOR THE VEGETABLE STEW

1 tablespoon coconut or avocado oil

2 garlic cloves, minced

½ onion, sliced lengthwise

Sea salt

1 bunch kale or mustard greens, stemmed and cut into 1-inch strips

1 summer squash, halved lengthwise and cut into half-moons

1 cup No-Mato sauce (page 122)

¼ cup coarsely chopped fresh cilantro

FOR THE MOFONGO

1 to 2 cups coconut oil, for frying

3 green/unripe plantains

4 garlic cloves, minced

Sea salt

2 tablespoons extra-virgin olive oil

TO MAKE THE VEGETABLE STEW

1. In a large saucepan over medium heat, warm the oil. Add the garlic, onion, and a pinch of salt. Cook for about 2 minutes, until the onion is translucent.

2. Add the kale and another pinch of salt. Cook until wilted, about 2 minutes. Add the squash, stir, and cook for 2 minutes.

3. Add the no-mato sauce and cilantro. Bring to a simmer, then cook for 3 to 5 minutes, until the flavors meld and the vegetables are tender. Set aside on a very low burner or turn off and reheat before serving.

TO MAKE THE MOFONGO

4. In a deep cast-iron pan, heat about 1 inch of oil to 350°F.

5. While the oil is heating, peel and slice the plantains into 1-inch rounds. Add them to the oil and fry for 5 to 7 minutes, until golden and tender. Transfer to paper towels to drain.

6. Using a mortar and pestle, mash the garlic and a pinch of salt into a paste.

7. In a large bowl or food processor, combine the plantains, olive oil, and garlic paste and mash until thoroughly blended, stiff, and slightly chunky, like mashed potatoes.

8. Shape the mofongo by separating the mash into 4 equal balls and pressing them into the bottom of small bowls, smoothing over, and inverting onto plates. Surround the mofongo with hot stew, then serve.

PER SERVING: Calories: 642; Total fat: 32g; Carbohydrates: 86g; Fiber: 8g; Protein: 6g; Sodium: 327mg

SWEET POTATO GNOCCHI WITH MUSHROOMS AND KALE

30 MINUTES OR LESS   COMFORT FOOD   VEGAN
Serves 2 / **Prep time:** 20 minutes / **Cook time:** 10 minutes

If you've never had gnocchi, you're in for a treat. They are a pillowy-soft, pasta-like dish traditionally made with potato. Making gnocchi requires a bit of effort, but the payoff is huge.

½ cup sweet potato puree

¾ cup whole cassava flour

¾ teaspoon sea salt, divided, plus 1 tablespoon

¼ cup water

1 tablespoon avocado oil

1 tablespoon sage leaves

3 garlic cloves, minced

1 shallot, minced

½ bunch kale, stemmed and chopped into bite-size pieces

6 to 8 cremini mushrooms, sliced

¼ cup no-bone broth (see Substitution tip, page 128)

1. In a large bowl, combine the sweet potato puree, cassava flour, and ½ teaspoon of salt. Add half the water, using your hands to combine the ingredients. Add more water as necessary to get a soft, pliable dough. Roll it into a ball.

2. Bring a large pot of water to a boil over high heat. Add 1 tablespoon of salt.

3. Meanwhile, cut the dough ball into 4 pieces using a pastry cutter or knife. On a dry work surface, roll each piece into a ½-inch-thick rope. Using the pastry cutter or knife, cut the dough into 1-inch pieces. Using a fork, lightly press grooves into each piece of gnocchi. Repeat this process with the other ropes.

4. Working in two batches, put half of the gnocchi into the boiling water. Cook for about 1 minute or until the gnocchi float to the top. Use a slotted spoon to transfer them to a large plate in a single layer.

5. Heat a large skillet over medium heat. Add the oil and sage leaves. Cook for about 30 seconds, until the leaves are crispy. Remove and set aside.

6. Add the garlic and shallot to the skillet and cook for about 30 seconds or until fragrant. Add the kale, the mushrooms, and the remaining ¼ teaspoon of salt and cook for 3 to 4 minutes, until the mushrooms are soft, the kale is wilted, and the pan is mostly dry.

7. Add the broth, stirring to get any browned bits off the bottom of the skillet. Cook for 2 to 3 minutes, until reduced by about half. Add the reserved gnocchi and stir to reheat, about 2 minutes. Top with the sage and serve.

MAKE-AHEAD TIP: Gnocchi can easily be made in large batches. Spread them out on a rimmed baking sheet and freeze for 30 to 45 minutes, until the outside is mostly frozen. Transfer to a freezer bag or freezer-safe container.

PER SERVING: Calories: 304; Total fat: 8g; Carbohydrates: 58g; Fiber: 7g; Protein: 5g; Sodium: 4,736mg

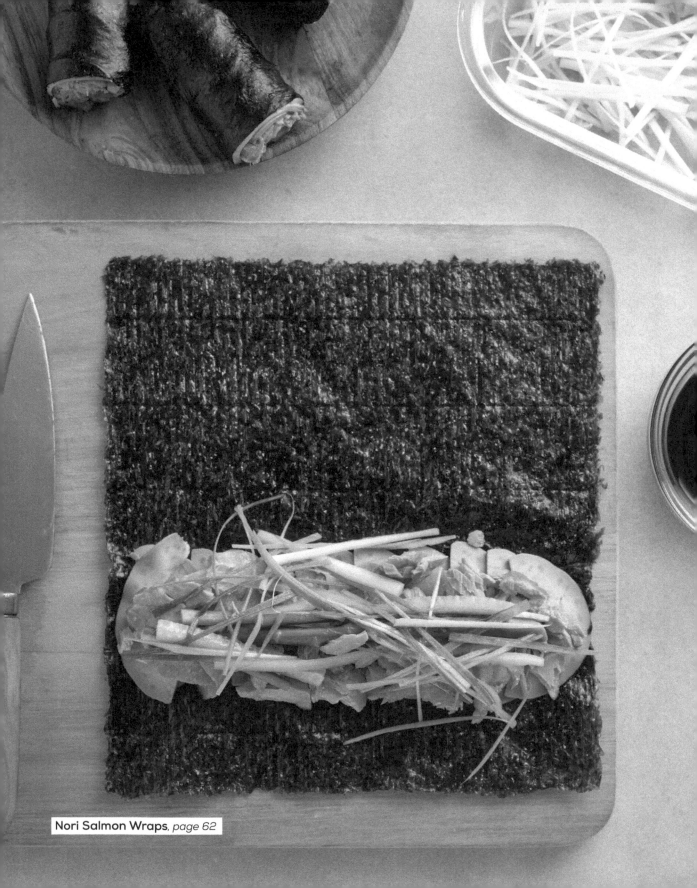

Nori Salmon Wraps, *page 62*

CHAPTER 5

SEAFOOD MAINS

LEMON AND DILL
POACHED SALMON WITH ASPARAGUS

30 MINUTES OR LESS   **ONE-POT MEAL**

Serves 2 / **Prep time:** 10 minutes / **Cook time:** 15 minutes

Shallow poaching under a piece of parchment paper, called a *cartouche*, in a pan is a quick way to get tender, flavorful fish while retaining all the great nutrients. Serve with a salad, cassava rice, or roasted butternut squash.

2 (6-ounce) Alaskan salmon fillets, skin on or removed

½ teaspoon sea salt, plus a pinch

3 tablespoons extra-virgin olive oil, divided

1 lemon, thinly sliced, reserving ½ inch of end

1 leek, halved lengthwise and thinly sliced

½ pound asparagus, woody ends removed, cut into 2-inch lengths

2 tablespoons chopped fresh dill, divided

¼ cup broth or water

¼ cup Coconut Yogurt (page 121)

1. Preheat the oven to 450°F. Sprinkle the salmon fillets with ½ teaspoon of salt. Measure a piece of parchment paper slightly larger than a large ovenproof skillet. Fold it in half from the bottom to the top, then left to right to form a square. Fold from one corner to form a triangle. Set one point of the parchment in the center of the skillet and mark the arc along the squared edge. Trim along the mark. Cut ½ inch off the folded end point. Unfold your cartouche and set it aside.

2. In the skillet you used to measure the parchment paper, over medium-high heat, warm 2 tablespoons of oil. Add the lemon slices and cook for 1 minute on each side. Add the leek and asparagus. Cook, stirring occasionally, for 4 to 5 minutes, until the leek is wilted. Add 1 tablespoon of dill and arrange the fillets in the mixture. Add the broth and top the skillet with the cartouche.

3. Bring the liquid to a simmer, then carefully transfer the skillet to the oven. Roast for 5 to 7 minutes, until the fillets are opaque and flaky.

4. Meanwhile, in a small bowl, whisk together the remaining 1 tablespoon of oil, the yogurt, and the lemon juice squeezed from the reserved end until emulsified to a mayonnaise-like consistency. Whisk in the remaining pinch of salt and the remaining 1 tablespoon of dill.

5. Remove the skillet from the oven. Transfer the fillets to a warm plate and cover with the cartouche. Set the skillet over medium heat. Bring the pan juices to a simmer and reduce slightly. Make sure the asparagus is fully cooked. Taste and add salt as needed. Remove from the heat.

6. Plate the fillets, topping with the asparagus mixture and a dollop of sauce. Serve immediately.

INGREDIENT TIP: Buy wild Alaskan salmon. It is a protected resource in that state, which ensures you are receiving pure, nutrient-dense fish. Farmed salmon have fewer omega-3 fatty acids and often contain artificial coloring.

PER SERVING: Calories: 526; Total fat: 34g; Carbohydrates: 14g; Fiber: 4g; Protein: 41g; Sodium: 850mg

COCONUT CLAM CHOWDER
WITH LEMONGRASS

30 MINUTES OR LESS   COMFORT FOOD
Serves 4 / **Prep time:** 10 minutes / **Cook time:** 20 minutes

This clam chowder is thickened with cassava instead of a flour roux. Coconut milk is used to get the richness, which is boosted with Thai-inspired flavors.

3 cups chicken Bone Broth (page 128)

1 lemongrass stalk, smashed slightly and cut into 2-inch lengths

20 littleneck clams

2 cups cubed cassava root or parsnip

3 uncured/nitrate-free bacon slices, halved lengthwise and cut into ½-inch batons

2 celery stalks, cut on the bias into ¼-inch slices

2 garlic cloves, minced

1 fennel bulb, cored and thinly sliced crosswise

1 onion, diced

1 (14-ounce) can coconut milk (no gums or carrageenan)

2 tablespoons coconut aminos

Juice of 1 lime

½ teaspoon sea salt

1 tablespoon chopped fresh cilantro

1 tablespoon chopped fresh Thai basil (optional)

1. In a large pot over medium-high heat, combine the broth and lemongrass and bring them to a simmer. Add the clams, cover, and cook for 5 to 7 minutes, until the clams open. Discard any clams that do not open. Remove the clams from their shells and coarsely chop. Set aside.

2. Add the cassava and cook for 7 to 10 minutes, until tender.

3. Meanwhile, in a large saucepan over medium heat, cook the bacon, stirring occasionally, for 5 to 7 minutes, until mostly rendered. Reserve the bacon pieces and set aside.

4. Add the celery, garlic, fennel, and onion to the bacon fat and cook, stirring, for 2 to 4 minutes, until the onion is translucent. Transfer everything to the pot. Add the clams, coconut milk, coconut aminos, and lime juice, and bring to a simmer.

5. Remove and discard the lemongrass. Add the salt. Garnish with the cilantro and basil (if using) and serve.

PER SERVING: Calories: 501; Total fat: 23g; Carbohydrates: 58g; Fiber: 6g; Protein: 20g; Sodium: 1,042mg

GRILLED HALIBUT WITH LEMON CAPER DRESSING

30 MINUTES OR LESS **ONE-POT MEAL**

Serves 2 / **Prep time:** 10 minutes / **Cook time:** 15 minutes

Cooking the fish on the grill gives it an extra burst of flavor and elevates the dish. If you can't grill, panfrying in a hot pan or under the broiler works, too. Serve this dish with a salad, grilled asparagus, artichokes, or Brussels sprouts.

½ to 1 pound halibut fillet, halved

1 lemon, halved

4 tablespoons extra-virgin olive oil, divided

1 tablespoon chopped fresh parsley

1 teaspoon granulated onion

½ teaspoon sea salt, plus a pinch

1 teaspoon chopped fresh dill

1 tablespoon capers

1. Prepare a grill to high heat. Brush the halibut and lemon with 1 tablespoon of oil. In a small bowl, combine the parsley, onion, and ½ teaspoon of salt. Sprinkle the mixture on both sides of the fish, then wipe out the bowl.

2. Put the lemon halves, cut-side down, on the grill for 2 to 5 minutes, until caramelized. Remove from the grill and, when cool enough to squeeze, juice into the small bowl. Add the remaining pinch of salt, the dill, and the remaining 3 tablespoons of oil, whisking until emulsified. Add the capers.

3. Place the halibut on the grill and cook for 3 minutes. Flip and cook for 3 to 5 minutes or until the flesh is opaque and firm.

4. Transfer the fish to a plate and top with the lemon caper sauce.

INGREDIENT TIP: Choose a center-cut fillet of halibut that is at least 1½ to 2 inches thick. Look for a bright white color and no fishy smell.

. . . .

PER SERVING: Calories: 357; Total fat: 29g; Carbohydrates: 4g; Fiber: 1g; Protein: 22g; Sodium: 765mg

HERB-BATTERED FISH AND CHIPS

30 MINUTES OR LESS COMFORT FOOD

Serves 2 / **Prep time:** 15 minutes / **Cook time:** 15 minutes

This dish feels like a real treat when you have eliminated so many things from your diet. The fresh herbs add a punch of flavor.

2 cups avocado or coconut oil, plus 1 tablespoon

1 cassava, peeled and cut into 5-inch sections

Sea salt

½ cup whole cassava flour

1 tablespoon chopped fresh herbs of choice

¼ cup water

½ pound whitefish, such as halibut, cut into 2-inch-wide strips

¼ cup tapioca starch

1. Place a rimmed baking sheet in the oven and preheat it to 500°F on the convection setting, if available. Heat 2 cups of oil in a deep cast-iron pan to 375°F.

2. Cut the cassava into ½-inch-thick planks, then halve the planks lengthwise. In a large bowl, combine the cassava, the remaining 1 tablespoon of oil, and salt to taste.

3. Open the oven and use tongs to put the cassava on the hot baking sheet, spacing it out as much as possible. Bake for 10 minutes, flip, and cook for 5 minutes more or until browning and tender.

4. In a large bowl, mix together the cassava flour, herbs, water, and a big pinch of salt. Add water as necessary to get a pancake-batter consistency. In a medium bowl, season the fish pieces with salt and coat with the tapioca starch.

5. Working in batches while the cassava roasts, dunk the fish pieces in the batter, then carefully add them to the hot oil. Cook for 3 minutes, flip, and cook for 3 more minutes. Transfer to a rack over paper towels to drain. Repeat for the remaining fish.

6. Remove the cassava fries from the oven and toss in a bowl with a little salt. Serve on a plate with the fish.

PER SERVING: Calories: 651; Total fat: 9g; Carbohydrates: 118g; Fiber: 6g; Protein: 24g; Sodium: 110mg

NIÇOISE SALAD WITH GRILLED FISH

30 MINUTES OR LESS   ONE-POT MEAL

Serves 2 / **Prep time:** 15 minutes / **Cook time:** 10 minutes

Typically, Niçoise salad is made with tuna. Because tuna has a high mercury content, we use grilled fish such as salmon, black cod, rockfish, or halibut. You can also use traditionally smoked salmon that has no additives.

8 ounces boneless, skinless fish, cut into 2 fillets

¼ cup extra-virgin olive oil, plus 1 tablespoon

Sea salt

2 garlic cloves, minced and mashed with salt

Juice of 1 lemon

5 to 8 fresh basil leaves, rolled and cut into thin ribbons

½ head butter lettuce, cut into 2-inch pieces

½ cup cremini mushrooms

6 cooked and cooled asparagus spears

½ avocado, sliced

½ cucumber, cut into ¼-inch slices

½ cup mixed olives, pitted

1. Prepare a grill to high heat or heat a broiler. Brush the fish with 1 tablespoon of oil and season with salt on both sides.

2. Put the fish on the grill and cook for 3 minutes. Flip and cook for 3 to 5 minutes or until the fish is just cooked through. Remove and set aside under a lid to stay warm.

3. In a small bowl, whisk together the remaining ¼ cup of oil, the mashed garlic, lemon juice, basil, and a pinch of salt. Toss the lettuce with half of the dressing, then split between two plates.

4. Toss the mushrooms and asparagus with the other half of the dressing and a pinch of salt. Add to the lettuce. Arrange the avocado and cucumber on top and season again with salt. Add the olives, top with the grilled fish, and pour any remaining dressing over the fish. Serve.

PER SERVING: Calories: 552; Total fat: 45g; Carbohydrates: 17g; Fiber: 5g; Protein: 27g; Sodium: 390mg

NORI SALMON WRAPS

30 MINUTES OR LESS **ONE-POT MEAL**

Serves 1 / **Prep time:** 20 minutes

Sometimes you just need a grab-and-go meal. Think of nori as an easy way to make a wrap that can enclose all kinds of fillings—cooked fish, vegetables, baby greens. Make them even more sushi-like with cauliflower rice.

3 nori sheets

½ avocado, thinly sliced

5 ounces salmon, pin bones removed, cooked and cooled

3 asparagus spears, cooked and cooled

½ cucumber, peeled and cut lengthwise twice into long strips

1 scallion, green part only, thinly sliced

2 tablespoons coconut aminos, divided

Sea salt

1. Lay one nori sheet on a cutting board with a long side toward you. Add a layer of avocado across the lower third of the sheet, leaving a narrow border. Top with one-third of the salmon, then add one-third of the asparagus and the cucumber strips. Top with some scallion, 1 teaspoon of coconut aminos, and a pinch of salt.

2. Roll by pulling the border over the filling and pulling toward you to tighten the filling in the roll. Continue to roll tightly until the sheet is nearly done. Wipe wet fingers along the edge of the nori to help seal and finish.

3. Repeat for the remaining sheets, being careful not to overstuff the rolls. Cut the rolls in half and serve with the remaining 1 tablespoon of coconut aminos for dipping.

MAKE-AHEAD TIP: Nori rolls will keep overnight, covered in the refrigerator, but much more time and they will start to get soggy.

PER SERVING: Calories: 336; Total fat: 12g; Carbohydrates: 23g; Fiber: 10g; Protein: 35g; Sodium: 650mg

SAFFRON SCALLOP PASTA WITH ARTICHOKES

Serves 2 / Prep time: 10 minutes / **Cook time:** 30 minutes

Scallop pasta with artichokes is spring on a plate and can be embellished with other spring vegetables, such as zucchini, fennel, and asparagus. Saffron is a powerful antioxidant with anti-inflammatory properties that adds a unique and exotic flavor to this dish.

2 artichokes, or 1 (12-ounce) jar artichoke hearts

½ (14-ounce) package cassava pasta, or spiralized zucchini

1 tablespoon avocado oil

½ pound sea scallops, dry (not packed in water) if available

½ teaspoon sea salt, plus more

2 shallots, chopped

2 garlic cloves, chopped

1 cup Bone Broth (page 128)

Pinch saffron threads

Juice of ½ lemon

. . . .

PER SERVING: Calories: 262; Total fat: 9g; Carbohydrates: 23g; Fiber: 10g; Protein: 22g; Sodium: 1,152mg

1. Chop the top off each artichoke and prepare a steamer. Place the artichokes in the steamer and cook for about 30 minutes. Transfer them to an ice bath, then peel the leaves from the hearts. Remove the center chokes. Dice the hearts and set aside.

2. Meanwhile, bring a large pot of water to a boil over high heat. Add the pasta and cook according to the package instructions until tender, usually about 10 minutes. Drain and set aside.

3. In a large skillet over medium-high heat, warm the oil. Dry the scallops with a paper towel and sprinkle with the salt. Carefully place the scallops in the skillet and cook for 1 to 2 minutes per side, until each side has a brown crust. Remove from the skillet and set aside.

4. Add the shallots and garlic to the skillet and cook until fragrant, about 30 seconds. Add the broth and deglaze the skillet by scraping the bottom. Bring to a simmer and reduce the broth slightly, for about 1 minute. Crush the saffron and add it to the broth along with the lemon juice. Season with salt.

5. Add the pasta, artichokes, and scallops to the sauce and toss with tongs. Plate and serve.

SALMON BURGERS WITH BAKED SWEET POTATOES

WORTH THE WAIT

Serves 2 / Prep time: 5 minutes / Cook time: 45 minutes

Salmon burgers are a great way to get more fish—packed with nutrients and important omega-3s—into your diet.

- **2 white sweet potatoes**
- **1 (½-pound) salmon fillet, skinned, pin bones removed, and cubed**
- **1 tablespoon Eggless Mayo (page 125)**
- **Juice of ½ lemon**
- **1 scallion, green and white parts, chopped**
- **1 tablespoon chopped fresh parsley**
- **½ tablespoon chopped fresh dill**
- **½ teaspoon sea salt, plus more for dressing and serving**
- **¼ cup whole cassava flour**
- **1 tablespoon avocado oil**
- **½ teaspoon extra-virgin olive oil, plus more for serving**
- **¼ teaspoon balsamic vinegar**
- **1 cup arugula or spring mix**

1. Preheat the oven to 450°F. Pierce the sweet potatoes with a fork. Put them on a rimmed baking sheet and roast for 45 minutes, until a knife pierces them easily.

2. Meanwhile, in a food processor, combine the salmon, mayo, lemon juice, scallion, parsley, dill, and salt. Pulse until the mixture is chopped and well combined. Add the cassava flour and mix thoroughly. Form into two ½- to ¾-inch-thick patties.

3. In a large, heavy skillet over medium heat, heat the avocado oil. Add the patties and cook for about 5 minutes on each side, until browned and opaque all the way through.

4. Meanwhile, in a medium bowl, whisk together the olive oil, vinegar, and salt to taste. Add the arugula and toss to coat. Transfer to two plates and top with the salmon burgers. Serve hot with the baked sweet potato drizzled with olive oil and salt.

MAKE-AHEAD TIP: Cook the sweet potatoes in advance and store them in the refrigerator, ready to be reheated in a 400°F oven for 15 to 20 minutes. Make a big batch of burgers in advance, then store, separated with wax paper, in the refrigerator.

. . . .

PER SERVING: Calories: 398; Total fat: 13g; Carbohydrates: 41g; Fiber: 4g; Protein: 27g; Sodium: 935mg

SHRIMP FRIED RICE

30 MINUTES OR LESS

Serves 2 / **Prep time:** 10 minutes / **Cook time:** 15 minutes

Fried rice is a delicious meal you can make in no time. Start with cooked cauliflower or cassava rice and precut vegetables from the refrigerator, and you can be eating shrimp fried rice faster than you can get takeout.

2 uncured/nitrate-free bacon slices, halved and cut into batons

1 (½-pound) large shrimp, peeled and deveined

Sea salt

2 tablespoons coconut aminos, divided

2 celery stalks, diced

2 garlic cloves, minced

1 carrot, diced

½ onion, diced

1 teaspoon minced fresh ginger

1 scallion, green and white parts separated, cut into rounds

1 tablespoon avocado or coconut oil

2 cups leftover cooled cauliflower or cassava rice

1. In a wok or large skillet over medium heat, cook the bacon, stirring occasionally, for 5 to 7 minutes, until mostly rendered. Transfer the bacon to paper towels to drain.

2. In the same wok, cook the shrimp with a pinch of salt, stirring frequently, for 2 minutes. Add 1 teaspoon of coconut aminos and cook, stirring, for another 1 minute, until the shrimp are no longer pink. Add the celery, garlic, carrot, onion, ginger, and scallion whites and cook, stirring frequently, for about 3 minutes, until the carrots are tender but not soft. Transfer the veggie-shrimp mixture to a bowl.

3. Heat the oil in the wok, add the cauliflower rice, and stir-fry for 30 seconds. Return the veggie-shrimp mix and bacon to the wok. Add the remaining 1 tablespoon of coconut aminos and cook, stirring, for 1 minute to reheat.

4. Taste and add salt or coconut aminos as needed. Serve in a bowl and garnish with the scallion greens.

MAKE-AHEAD TIP: Precut the vegetables and store in the refrigerator.

SUBSTITUTION TIP: There are brands making a cassava orzo, which is rice-shaped pasta that would work nicely in this recipe in place of the rice.

PER SERVING: Calories: 262; Total fat: 10g; Carbohydrates: 17g; Fiber: 5g; Protein: 25g; Sodium: 645mg

SHRIMP TACOS WITH PLANTAIN TORTILLAS AND CILANTRO LIME SLAW

WORTH THE WAIT

Serves 2 / Prep time: 20 minutes / Cook time: 30 minutes

Plantain tortillas are a great alternative to corn or flour tortillas and go well with pork, shredded beef, fish, or this garlicky shrimp. topped with a bright lime cilantro slaw.

FOR THE TORTILLAS

1 green plantain, peeled and chopped

2 tablespoons whole cassava flour, plus more for shaping

Pinch sea salt

1 teaspoon avocado oil

FOR THE TACOS

¼ cup Eggless Mayo (page 125)

½ cup chopped scallions, green and white parts

¼ cup chopped fresh cilantro

Juice of 2 limes, divided

2 garlic cloves, minced

Sea salt

2 cups shredded green cabbage

½ cup shredded red cabbage

1 tablespoon avocado oil

1 pound wild shrimp, peeled and deveined, tails removed

½ avocado, mashed

TO MAKE THE TORTILLAS

1. In a medium pot of boiling water, cook the plantain for 15 minutes, until soft. Transfer the plantain to a food processor. Add the cassava flour, salt, and oil. Process until a dough ball forms. It should be soft but a bit tacky.

2. Flour your hands with cassava flour and divide the dough into 6 equal balls. Place one dough ball between two lightly oiled sheets of parchment paper and gently start to press it down with your hands, creating a circle of dough underneath. Use a rolling pin to roll out a 5-inch tortilla about ⅛-inch thick. Leave it between the parchment paper sheets and set aside. Repeat with the remaining dough balls.

3. Heat a medium cast-iron skillet over medium heat. Working with one tortilla at a time, peel off one side of the parchment and flip the tortilla over to lay the uncovered side in the skillet. Cook for 1 to 2 minutes, remove the top parchment, and flip, then cook for 1 to 2 more minutes, until brown blisters form. Set aside. Repeat with the remaining tortillas.

TO MAKE THE TACOS

1. In a large bowl, whisk together the mayo, scallions, cilantro, the juice of 1 lime, a pinch of garlic, and a pinch of salt. Add the green and red cabbage and toss to combine.

2. In a large skillet over medium-high heat, warm the oil. Add the shrimp and cook for 1 to 2 minutes per side, until the shrimp are opaque. Add the remaining garlic and mix well. Remove from the heat, add the remaining lime juice, and season with salt. Stir.

3. To assemble, spread an equal amount of avocado over each tortilla. Fill each with shrimp and top with slaw. Serve.

INGREDIENT TIP: You can use cassava tortillas (page 132) in place of the plantain tortillas.

MAKE-AHEAD TIP: Make tortillas ahead of time and keep a stash in the refrigerator. Reheat in a hot pan for 15 to 20 seconds per side. This cuts the time to make the recipe to about 15 minutes.

PER SERVING (3 TACOS): Calories: 733; Total fat: 28g; Carbohydrates: 71g; Fiber: 9g; Protein: 52g; Sodium: 356mg

THAI-STYLE WHITEFISH CURRY

30 MINUTES OR LESS

Serves 2 / **Prep time:** 15 minutes / **Cook time:** 15 minutes

This coconut-based curry is perfect for a whitefish, such as cod or halibut. Though Thai food is known for being spicy, the cuisine balances sweet, hot, salty, sour, and bitter flavors. I have left out the heat here for the elimination phase, but horseradish could be added. Serve over cauliflower or cassava rice, yam (glass or shirataki) noodles, or grain-free cassava spaghetti noodles.

1 (14-ounce) can coconut milk (no gums or carrageenan)

1 lemongrass stalk, smashed slightly and cut into 2-inch lengths

2 tablespoons coconut aminos

½ teaspoon ground turmeric

6 garlic cloves, minced

2 tablespoons avocado or coconut oil

2 shallots, thinly sliced

1 teaspoon grated fresh ginger

½ pound broccoli, bok choy, spinach, or kale, chopped into bite-size pieces

1 (½-pound) firm whitefish, cut into 2-inch cubes

Juice of 1 lime

½ teaspoon sea salt

1 tablespoon chopped fresh cilantro

1 tablespoon chopped fresh Thai or Italian basil

1 teaspoon chopped fresh mint

1. In a large saucepan over medium-high heat, combine the coconut milk, lemongrass, coconut aminos, turmeric, and a third of the garlic and bring to a simmer. Reduce the heat to low to maintain a gentle simmer, not a boil.

2. In a wok or large skillet over medium-high heat, warm the oil. Add the shallots and cook, stirring frequently, for 1 minute, until slightly browned. Add the ginger and the remaining two-thirds of the garlic, stirring until fragrant, about 30 seconds. Add the broccoli and stir-fry for 2 to 3 minutes, until it starts to cook down.

3. Transfer the simmering curry sauce to the wok along with the fish, lime juice, salt, cilantro, basil, and mint. Bring back to a simmer and cook for 5 to 7 minutes, until the broccoli is soft and the fish is cooked through. Taste and add salt as needed, then serve.

INGREDIENT TIP: If you are using cassava noodles, bring a large pot of water to a boil, and cook according to the instructions on the package. Try to time the pasta being done (usually 10 minutes) to the fish being fully cooked so everything is hot.

PER SERVING: Calories: 633; Total fat: 49g; Carbohydrates: 29g; Fiber: 6g; Protein: 27g; Sodium: 1,021mg

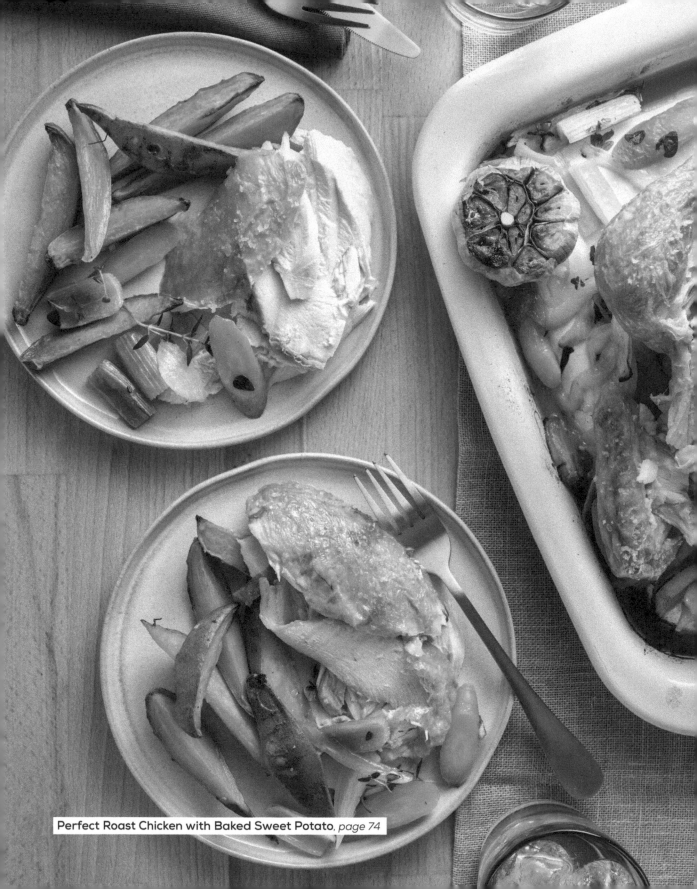

Perfect Roast Chicken with Baked Sweet Potato, *page 74*

CHAPTER 6

POULTRY MAINS

TURKEY BURGERS WITH BUTTERNUT SQUASH HASH

Serves 2 / Prep time: 10 minutes / **Cook time:** 30 minutes

These turkey burgers are inspired by the work done by the people of *America's Test Kitchen*, who found that adding gelatin to the turkey burger keeps it moist and baking soda raises the pH, changing the protein structure to better hold moisture and brown more evenly. The butternut squash and apple hash make a perfect fall complement to our herbed turkey burger.

2 cups butternut squash, cut into 1-inch cubes

½ tablespoon avocado oil, plus 1 teaspoon

½ teaspoon sea salt, plus a pinch

4 uncured/nitrate-free bacon slices, cut into lardons

½ large onion, diced

1 large apple, peeled and chopped

½ pound ground turkey thigh

1 teaspoon pasture-raised gelatin, bloomed in 2 tablespoons water

½ teaspoon dried ground sage

½ teaspoon minced fresh oregano

½ teaspoon minced fresh thyme

¼ teaspoon baking soda

1. Preheat the oven to 450°F. Line a rimmed baking sheet with parchment paper.

2. On the prepared baking sheet, toss together the squash, ½ tablespoon of oil, and a pinch of salt to coat, then spread out evenly. Bake for 30 minutes, until the edges of the squash are browned and starting to crisp.

3. Meanwhile, in a large skillet over medium heat, cook the bacon, stirring occasionally, for 5 to 7 minutes, until mostly rendered. Transfer the bacon to paper towels to drain. In the same skillet with the bacon fat, cook the onion for about 2 minutes, until translucent. Add the apple and cook, stirring frequently, for 2 minutes. Transfer to a large bowl and set aside.

4. In a large bowl, combine the turkey, bloomed gelatin, sage, oregano, thyme, baking soda, and the remaining ½ teaspoon of salt. Mix thoroughly with your hands and form into 2 patties.

5. Wipe the large skillet clean, pour in the remaining 1 teaspoon of oil, and set it over medium-high heat until sizzling hot. Add the turkey burgers and cook for 5 to 6 minutes, or until they are browned and release easily from the skillet. Flip and cook for another 4 to 5 minutes, until they are firm and an instant-read thermometer reads 165°F when inserted into the center. Remove from the skillet and let rest for 2 minutes.

6. Add the roasted squash and bacon to the apple-onion mixture, tossing to combine. Serve on a plate with the turkey burger.

PER SERVING: Calories: 438; Total fat: 24g; Carbohydrates: 32g; Fiber: 7g; Protein: 28g; Sodium: 1,085mg

PERFECT ROAST CHICKEN WITH BAKED SWEET POTATO

COMFORT FOOD   WORTH THE WAIT

Serves 2 / **Prep time:** 10 minutes / **Cook time:** 1 hour 30 minutes

Few things are more delicious than a perfectly roasted chicken—a vessel for nearly any type of meal and flavoring you can imagine. After you eat, use the carcass to make Bone Broth (page 128).

1 (5-pound) whole chicken, giblets removed, rinsed, and patted dry

2 tablespoons extra-virgin olive oil, divided

Sea salt

1 bunch fresh thyme

1 leek, quartered

1 garlic bulb, top third of cloves chopped off

1 lemon or apple, stemmed, seeded, and halved

1 large yellow onion, thickly sliced

4 carrots, cut into large chunks

4 celery stalks, cut into large chunks

2 sweet potatoes

Olive oil or coconut oil, for serving

1. Set a roasting pan just large enough to hold the chicken in the oven and preheat it to 425°F.

2. Rub the chicken with 1 tablespoon of oil and season all over with salt. Set a few thyme sprigs aside, then stuff the rest in the cavity. Add the leek, garlic, and lemon to the cavity. Tie the end of the legs together with kitchen twine and tuck the wing tips under the bird.

3. In a large bowl, toss together the onion, carrots, celery, a large pinch of salt, the remaining 1 tablespoon of oil, and the reserved thyme. Carefully pour the vegetables into the preheated roasting pan, spreading them around. Put the chicken on top. Roast for 1½ hours or until the juices run clear between the leg and thigh and an instant-read thermometer registers 155°F in the breast and 170°F in the thigh.

4. Meanwhile, poke the sweet potatoes all over with a fork and put in a small ovenproof pan. Start roasting the potatoes after the chicken has been cooking for 30 minutes. Roast for about 1 hour, until tender.

5. When the chicken is done, remove it from the pan, cover with aluminum foil or the pan lid, and let sit for 15 minutes.

6. Slice the chicken and arrange on a platter with the roasted vegetables. Drizzle oil over the baked sweet potatoes and serve.

INGREDIENT TIP: You'll have plenty of leftover chicken. Use it for a fast lunch with a salad or stuffed into plantain tortillas with avocado and a squeeze of lime.

. . . .

PER SERVING (4 OUNCES CHICKEN AND 1 POTATO): Calories: 588; Total fat: 29g; Carbohydrates: 58g; Fiber: 12g; Protein: 27g; Sodium: 315mg

COCONUT CHICKEN SOUP (TOM KHA GAI)

30 MINUTES OR LESS **ONE-POT MEAL** **VEGAN OPTION**

Serves 4 / **Prep time:** 10 minutes / **Cook time:** 20 minutes

Thailand's tom kha soup is packed with nutrients and fits into the AIP with little modification. Try serving this as a curry with cauliflower rice: Use 1 cup of stock and add vegetable or cassava noodles for a fast, nutritious dinner.

1 tablespoon coconut oil

1 shallot, cut into ¼-inch slices

3 garlic cloves, thinly sliced

3 cups Bone Broth (page 128)

1 (14-ounce) can coconut milk (no gums or carrageenan), cream separated and reserved

3 tablespoons fish sauce

2 lemongrass stalks, trimmed to 3 inches and smashed

1-inch piece fresh galangal or ginger, smashed

2 makrut lime leaves (or lime zest)

2 tablespoons chopped fresh cilantro

2 tablespoons Thai basil, cut into thin ribbons (optional)

½ teaspoon sea salt

½ pound skinless chicken breast, thinly sliced crosswise

½ cup shiitake mushrooms, thinly sliced (optional)

Juice of 1 lime

1. In a soup pot over medium heat, warm the oil and sauté the shallot and garlic for about 2 minutes, until the shallot is translucent. Add the broth, the liquid part of the coconut milk, the fish sauce, lemongrass, galangal, lime leaves, cilantro, basil (if using), and salt and bring to a simmer. Cook for 10 minutes.

2. Add the chicken and mushrooms (if using). Simmer for 10 minutes or until the chicken is fully cooked. Taste and add salt as needed.

3. Remove from the heat. Discard the galangal, lime leaves, and lemongrass and stir in the reserved coconut cream and lime juice. Serve.

INGREDIENT TIP: Boost your anti-inflammatory and gut-healing support by adding ¼ teaspoon of ground turmeric and/or ½ teaspoon each of turkey tail, reishi, and chaga mushroom powders.

SUBSTITUTION TIP: Make this vegan by omitting the chicken and using no-bone broth instead of bone broth and coconut aminos instead of fish sauce.

PER SERVING: Calories: 315; Total fat: 24g; Carbohydrates: 8g; Fiber: 1g; Protein: 18g; Sodium: 1,439mg

CHICKEN AND BROCCOLI STIR-FRY WITH WATER CHESTNUTS

30 MINUTES OR LESS   ONE-POT MEAL

Serves 2 / **Prep time:** 10 minutes / **Cook time:** 10 minutes

This classic stir-fry dish comes together quickly for a highly nutritious meal. Water chestnuts are high in potassium, manganese, and copper, as well as vitamin B_6—all components important for protein synthesis. Water chestnuts, broccoli, garlic, and ginger are also high in antioxidants.

1 tablespoon tapioca starch

¼ cup water

3 tablespoons avocado or coconut oil

2 teaspoons minced garlic

2 teaspoons minced fresh ginger

2 teaspoons sliced scallion, green and white parts separated

½ onion, cut into thin wedges

1 pound boneless, skinless chicken breast, cut into 1-inch dice

2 cups broccoli florets, blanched in salted water

½ cup water chestnuts

¼ cup coconut aminos

½ cup chicken Bone Broth (page 128)

Sea salt

Cauliflower or cassava rice, for serving

1. In a small bowl, combine the tapioca starch and water to create a slurry. Set aside.

2. In a wok or large skillet over high heat, warm the oil, swirling to coat the pan, until sizzling hot. Add the garlic, ginger, scallion whites, and onion, and stir-fry for 1 minute.

3. Add the chicken and stir-fry for 3 minutes, until browned. Stir in the broccoli and water chestnuts. Add the coconut aminos and cook until reduced slightly, about 30 seconds.

4. Add the broth and bring to a boil. Stir in the tapioca slurry. Reduce the heat and cook for 2 to 3 minutes, until thickened. Taste and add salt as needed. Serve over cauliflower rice and garnish with the scallion greens.

PER SERVING: Calories: 592; Total fat: 27g; Carbohydrates: 25g; Fiber: 5g; Protein: 57g; Sodium: 844mg

FRIED CHICKEN WITH SWEET POTATO WAFFLES

COMFORT FOOD

Serves 4 / **Prep time:** 10 minutes / **Cook time:** 25 minutes

Fried chicken is even better with a crisp and soft sweet potato waffle.
Top with your favorite AIP-compliant condiment, maple syrup, or Barbecue
Sauce (page 123).

FOR THE WAFFLES

1 cup whole cassava flour

1 scoop/serving grass-fed/
finished collagen peptides
(see Resources, page 140)

1 teaspoon ground cinnamon

1 teaspoon baking powder

¼ teaspoon baking soda

¼ teaspoon sea salt

¼ teaspoon ground ginger

1 cup sweet potato puree

2 tablespoons avocado oil

½ cup coconut milk (no
gums or carrageenan) or
water

TO MAKE THE WAFFLES

1. Preheat a waffle maker. Preheat the oven to 300°F.

2. In a large bowl, combine the cassava flour, collagen, cinnamon, baking powder, baking soda, salt, and ginger. In a separate bowl, whisk together the sweet potato puree and oil, then add to the flour mixture and mix until smooth, adding the coconut milk until you get a thick, pourable batter.

3. Pour batter onto the center of the waffle maker until three-fourths of the surface is covered. Close the waffle maker and cook for 3 minutes. Repeat with the remaining batter. Put finished waffles in the oven to stay warm.

TO MAKE THE CHICKEN

4. In a deep cast-iron pan over high heat, heat the oil to 375°F. Set a wire rack on a rimmed baking sheet.

5. In a large bowl, mix together the flour, thyme, oregano, celery salt, garlic, water, and salt. Add more water as necessary to get to a pancake-batter consistency.

FOR THE CHICKEN

2 cups avocado or
  coconut oil

1 cup whole cassava flour

½ teaspoon dried thyme

½ teaspoon dried oregano

½ teaspoon celery salt

½ teaspoon granulated
  garlic

½ cup water

½ teaspoon sea salt

1 pound boneless, skinless
  chicken breast, pounded
  to a uniform thickness

¼ cup tapioca starch

6. In a separate bowl, sprinkle the chicken pieces with salt and coat with the tapioca starch.

7. Working in batches to not overcrowd the pan, fry the chicken by dunking it into the batter, then carefully placing in the hot oil. Cook for 3 minutes, flip, then cook for 3 more minutes. Transfer to the prepared baking sheet and put into the warm oven.

8. Serve the fried chicken on the waffles.

MAKE-AHEAD TIP: Waffles can be made in advance, stored in the refrigerator, and reheated in a 300°F oven while you fry the chicken.

. . . .

PER SERVING: Calories: 618; Total fat: 22g; Carbohydrates: 74g; Fiber: 6g; Protein: 33g; Sodium: 1,021mg

POLLO ASADO FAJITA BOWLS

VEGAN OPTION

Serves 4 / **Prep time:** 10 minutes / **Cook time:** 25 minutes

Our fajitas are cooked on a single rimmed baking sheet in the oven to simplify preparation. This dish is served like a salad here but would be equally good stuffed into Cassava Tortillas (page 132).

2 teaspoons dried oregano

½ teaspoon sea salt

½ teaspoon ground ginger

½ teaspoon ground cinnamon

½ teaspoon ground turmeric

¼ cup avocado oil

Juice of 1 lime

1 pound boneless, skinless chicken, cut into strips

1 small onion, sliced lengthwise

1 small acorn, delicata, or summer squash, cut into half-moons

2 carrots, cut into strips

3 cups butter lettuce, green leaf, or spring mix lettuce

1 avocado, sliced

¼ cup sliced black olives

2 tablespoons chopped fresh cilantro

1 lime, cut into wedges

1. Preheat the oven to 400°F.

2. In a large bowl, combine the oregano, salt, ginger, cinnamon, and turmeric. Add the oil and lime juice and whisk until emulsified. Transfer two-thirds of the dressing to a small bowl.

3. Add the chicken to the large bowl with the remaining third of the dressing and mix until thoroughly coated. In a separate large bowl, combine the onion, squash, carrots, and half of the reserved dressing, tossing to coat.

4. Arrange the chicken and vegetables on a rimmed baking sheet, keeping the chicken separate to make it easier to remove the vegetables if they finish faster. Bake for 20 to 25 minutes, until the chicken registers 165°F on an instant-read thermometer and the vegetables are soft. Remove from the oven and let cool slightly.

5. Meanwhile, toss the lettuce with the remaining dressing and arrange in bowls. Top with the chicken and vegetables, avocado, black olives, and cilantro. Serve with lime wedges for squeezing.

SUBSTITUTION TIP: Omit the chicken for a vegan option.

PER SERVING: Calories: 378; Total fat: 23g; Carbohydrates: 16g; Fiber: 6g; Protein: 28g; Sodium: 523mg

CHICKEN SOUP

COMFORT FOOD ONE-POT MEAL WORTH THE WAIT

Serves 4 / **Prep time:** 15 minutes / **Cook time:** 35 minutes

The addition of No-Mato Sauce and spinach makes for a heartier soup than the chicken noodle of your childhood. The coconut milk adds richness, and the cassava flour helps thicken the soup slightly.

½ **pound boneless skinless chicken breast, cut into large dice**

2 **teaspoons sea salt, plus a pinch**

2 **tablespoons avocado oil, divided**

3 **celery stalks, diced**

2 **carrots, diced**

1 **onion, diced**

1 **tablespoon minced garlic**

½ **teaspoon dried thyme**

½ **teaspoon dried oregano**

8 **cups chicken Bone Broth (page 128)**

2 **cups No-Mato Sauce (page 122)**

1 **tablespoon whole cassava flour**

¼ **cup coconut milk (no gums or carrageenan) or water**

2 **cups fresh spinach, thinly sliced**

1. Season the chicken with 2 teaspoons of salt. Heat 1 tablespoon of oil in a large soup pot over medium-high heat. Add the chicken and cook, stirring occasionally, for about 3 minutes, until browned on all sides. Transfer the chicken to a plate.

2. Add the remaining 1 tablespoon of oil, the celery, carrots, and onion and cook for about 5 minutes, until the onion is translucent. Add the garlic, thyme, oregano, and a pinch of salt and cook until fragrant, about 15 seconds.

3. Add the broth and no-mato sauce and bring to a simmer. Cook for about 15 minutes, then mix the cassava flour with the coconut milk and add the slurry to the pot, stirring to combine.

4. Add the browned chicken and spinach, and simmer for another 10 minutes, until the soup has thickened and the chicken is cooked all the way through. Serve right away.

MAKE IT MILDER: Simplify the soup by leaving out the spinach and no-mato sauce. The soup will be brothy, but you can thicken it by blending the vegetables with the broth before returning the chicken to the pot.

PER SERVING: Calories: 468; Total fat: 31g; Carbohydrates: 23g; Fiber: 5g; Protein: 24g; Sodium: 1,915mg

CHICKEN TIKKA MASALA

WORTH THE WAIT

Serves 4 / **Prep time:** 10 minutes, plus 15 minutes to marinate
Cook time: 20 minutes

Chicken tikka masala, full of warming spices and a rich and tangy sauce, is one of the most popular Indian-inspired dishes outside of India. Stuff left-over chicken into plantain tortillas for a quick and delicious lunch.

2 teaspoons ground turmeric

1 teaspoon ground cinnamon

¼ teaspoon ground cloves

1 teaspoon sea salt, divided

1 pound skinless chicken thighs, cut into large dice

½ cup Coconut Yogurt (page 121)

½ onion, diced

3 garlic cloves, chopped

1-inch piece fresh ginger, chopped

¼ cup Bone Broth (page 128)

2 tablespoons avocado or coconut oil

1 cup No-Mato Sauce (page 122)

½ (14-ounce) can coconut milk (no gums or carrageenan)

¼ cup chopped fresh cilantro

2 scallions, green parts only, chopped

1. In a small bowl, combine the turmeric, cinnamon, cloves, and ½ teaspoon of salt. In a large bowl, combine the chicken with half the spice blend and the coconut yogurt. Marinate for 15 minutes to 1 hour.

2. In a food processor, pulse the onion, garlic, and ginger until well chopped. Add the broth and process to a wet paste.

3. In a large skillet over medium-high heat, warm the oil. Add the paste and sauté for 2 minutes, until it is fragrant and most of the liquid has evaporated. Add the remaining spice mix to the center of the skillet. When fragrant, stir to mix.

4. Add the chicken. Cook for 3 minutes, until browned. Add the no-mato sauce and coconut milk, scraping up any browned bits. Bring to a simmer and cook for 10 minutes, until the sauce thickens and deepens in color and the chicken is cooked through.

5. Taste and add the remaining ½ teaspoon of salt as needed. Garnish with the cilantro and scallions.

INGREDIENT TIP: Chicken breast can be used but would benefit from marinating longer. You can also replace the chicken with turkey, which offers a great amino acid profile for gut health.

PER SERVING: Calories: 438; Total fat: 34g; Carbohydrates: 15g; Fiber: 3g; Protein: 22g; Sodium: 1,060mg

ROASTED SAFFRON CHICKEN WITH STONE FRUIT

WORTH THE WAIT

Serves 4 / **Prep time:** 10 minutes, plus 1 hour to rest / **Cook time:** 50 minutes

Chicken roasted with fruit is shockingly delicious. Roasting the fruit with the chicken breaks down the fruit and makes a delightfully savory sauce—tart, sweet, and spicy. Prep the marinade the night before and marinate the chicken in a pan overnight to get even more flavor out of this dish, and save time!

3 garlic cloves, chopped

1 lemon, zested then quartered

2 teaspoons sea salt

½ teaspoon saffron threads

3 tablespoons extra-virgin olive oil, divided

2 pounds skin-on chicken thighs and legs

1 pound plums or apricots, cut into 1-inch slices

2 leeks, halved lengthwise then cut into half-moons

1 teaspoon grated fresh ginger

¼ teaspoon ground cinnamon

⅛ teaspoon ground cloves

½ teaspoon sea salt

4 bay leaves

1. Using a mortar and pestle, mash the garlic, lemon zest, salt, and saffron into a paste. Mix the paste with 2 tablespoons of oil. Rub the mixture all over the chicken and let sit for 1 hour.

2. Preheat the oven to 425°F.

3. In a large bowl, toss the plums with the lemon quarters, the remaining 1 tablespoon of oil, the leeks, ginger, cinnamon, cloves, and salt.

4. Arrange the chicken on a rimmed baking sheet or large roasting pan and spoon the fruit mixture around the chicken, filling in the gaps. Add the bay leaves to the mixture. Roast for 45 to 50 minutes, until the fruit has broken down, creating a sauce, and the chicken skin is browned and crisp. The chicken should register 165°F on an instant-read thermometer.

5. Remove the lemon and bay leaves and arrange the chicken on a platter. Serve with the fruit sauce spooned over the chicken.

PER SERVING: Calories: 658; Total fat: 39g; Carbohydrates: 21g; Fiber: 3g; Protein: 54g; Sodium: 1,668mg

BARBECUE CHICKEN WINGS WITH ROASTED BRUSSELS SPROUTS AND BACON

5 INGREDIENT   WORTH THE WAIT

Serves 2 / **Prep time:** 10 minutes / **Cook time:** 1 hour 5 minutes

The Barbecue Sauce makes these wings irresistible, and you won't feel as though you're missing out on anything. Double or triple the number of wings to have leftovers that are super easy to reheat and enjoy.

8 chicken wings, drumettes and wings

1 tablespoon avocado oil

1 teaspoon sea salt, divided

2 uncured/nitrate-free bacon slices, cut into lardons

½ pound Brussels sprouts

½ cup Barbecue Sauce (page 123), plus more for dipping, if needed

. . . .

PER SERVING: Calories: 477; Total fat: 32g; Carbohydrates: 20g; Fiber: 5g; Protein: 27g; Sodium: 1,857mg

1. Preheat the oven to 375°F.

2. In a large bowl, toss the chicken wings with the oil and ½ teaspoon of salt. Transfer to a rimmed baking sheet in a single layer, making sure not to crowd them. Bake for 50 to 60 minutes, until the wings are browned and crispy.

3. Meanwhile, in a large skillet over medium heat, cook the bacon, stirring occasionally, for 5 to 7 minutes, until mostly rendered. Transfer the bacon to paper towels to drain.

4. Trim the stems of the Brussels sprouts, discard any loose outer leaves, and cut in half. Put the sprouts in a roasting pan and pour the bacon fat over them. Add the remaining ½ teaspoon of salt and stir to mix. When the wings have about 45 minutes left, put the sprouts in the oven and roast for about 15 minutes, until dark and all the bacon fat has been absorbed.

5. Transfer the wings to a large stainless steel bowl. Toss with the barbecue sauce, then put them back on the baking sheet and return to the oven for 5 minutes to glaze the wings.

6. Stir the reserved bacon pieces into the sprouts. Serve with the wings and extra barbecue sauce, if desired.

CHICKEN TERIYAKI BOWL

30 MINUTES OR LESS   VEGETARIAN OPTION

Serves 2 / **Prep time:** 10 minutes / **Cook time:** 15 minutes

Coconut aminos really comes into its own in this teriyaki sauce, delivering an umami punch along with the blackstrap molasses. This bowl will keep you satisfied for hours.

FOR THE TERIYAKI SAUCE

½ cup coconut aminos

1 tablespoon honey

1 teaspoon garlic, chopped

1 teaspoon grated fresh ginger

¼ teaspoon sea salt

¼ teaspoon blackstrap molasses

1 tablespoon water

1 teaspoon arrowroot powder

FOR THE BOWL

2 tablespoons avocado oil, divided

1 onion, halved and sliced lengthwise

1 carrot, cut into thin strips

1 head broccoli, cut into small florets and blanched

¼ teaspoon sea salt

½ pound boneless, skinless chicken breast, cut into 1-inch cubes

2 cups cooked cauliflower or cassava rice

½ avocado, sliced

¼ cup crumbled nori sheets

TO MAKE THE TERIYAKI SAUCE

1. In a small saucepan over medium heat, combine the coconut aminos, honey, garlic, ginger, salt, and molasses and bring to a simmer. Combine the water and arrowroot powder to make a slurry, then add it to the sauce and cook until thickened, 2 to 3 minutes. Remove from the heat and let cool.

TO MAKE THE BOWL

2. In a wok or large skillet over high heat, warm 1 tablespoon of oil until sizzling hot. Add the onion, carrot, broccoli, and salt and stir-fry for 3 to 4 minutes. Transfer the veggies to a bowl.

3. Add the chicken to the wok with the remaining 1 tablespoon of oil and stir-fry for 3 to 4 minutes, until browned. Add 2 tablespoons of teriyaki sauce and cook for 1 minute, until glazed and cooked through. Add the chicken to the veggies. Add more teriyaki sauce and toss.

4. Divide the cauliflower rice between two bowls. Add the vegetables and chicken with more sauce, as desired. Top with the avocado and nori, and serve.

SUBSTITUTION TIP: Replace the chicken with chopped portobello mushrooms for a vegetarian version.

PER SERVING: Calories: 583; Total fat: 23g; Carbohydrates: 60g; Fiber: 15g; Protein: 39g; Sodium: 1,874mg

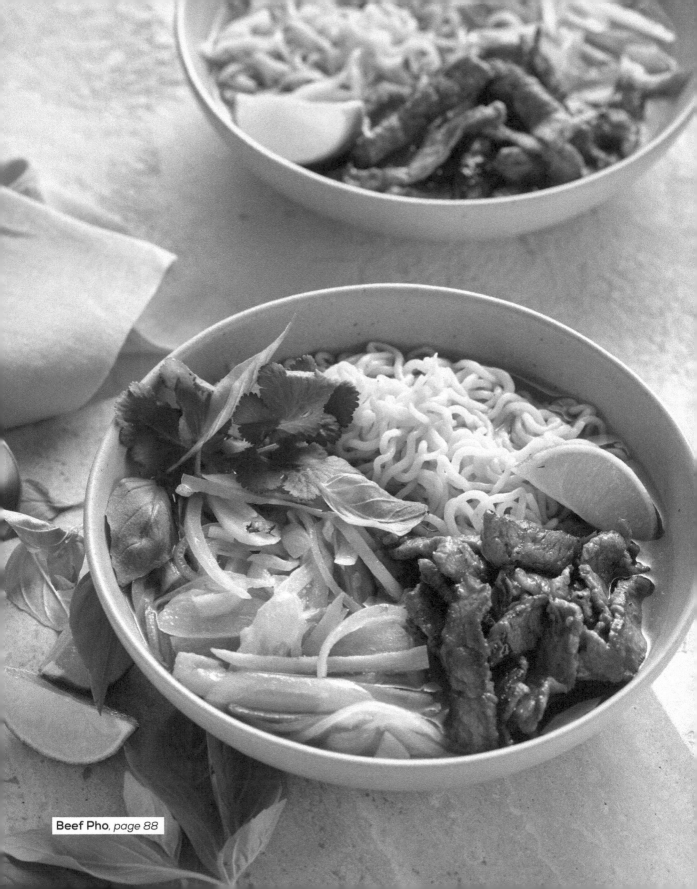

Beef Pho, *page 88*

CHAPTER 7

BEEF, PORK, AND LAMB MAINS

BEEF PHO

WORTH THE WAIT

Serves 2 / **Prep time:** 15 minutes / **Cook time:** 30 minutes

Pho is perhaps the world's greatest noodle soup and one of the best ways to use bone broth. The warm spice from the cinnamon and licorice notes from the fennel play well with the lime's citrus.

1 quart Bone Broth
(page 128)

1-inch piece fresh ginger, halved and smashed

6 garlic cloves, peeled, divided

1 large onion, halved lengthwise

2 cinnamon sticks or 1 teaspoon ground cinnamon

1 fennel bulb, halved, divided

2 teaspoons sea salt, divided

¼ cup fish sauce or coconut aminos

1 tablespoon avocado oil

½ pound beef sirloin, sliced across the grain as thinly as possible

1 package yam (glass or shirataki) noodles

¼ cup chopped fresh cilantro

Thai basil leaves, for serving

1 lime, cut into wedges

1. In a large pot over high heat, combine the bone broth, ginger, 3 garlic cloves, half the onion, the cinnamon, half the fennel, and 1 teaspoon of salt and bring to a boil. Cook for 30 minutes, then add the fish sauce. Taste and add the remaining 1 teaspoon of salt as needed.

2. Meanwhile, in a large skillet over medium heat, heat the oil. Cut the remaining onion and fennel halves lengthwise and chop the remaining 3 garlic cloves. Add everything to the skillet and cook, stirring frequently, for about 2 minutes, until the onion and fennel are translucent. Add the beef and cook for 1 to 2 minutes, until no longer pink. Be careful not to overcook the beef as it will get chewy.

3. Fill two bowls with the broth and add the noodles. Add the beef and vegetable mixture. Top with the cilantro and basil and serve with lime wedges.

MAKE-AHEAD TIP: Make a batch of pho broth from your bone broth and store in the refrigerator in a glass jar.

PER SERVING: Calories: 413; Total fat: 19g; Carbohydrates: 28g; Fiber: 7g; Protein: 38g; Sodium: 5,326mg

PORK CHOPS WITH SQUASH AND APPLES

30 MINUTES OR LESS COMFORT FOOD ONE-POT MEAL

Serves 2 / **Prep time:** 10 minutes / **Cook time:** 20 minutes

Pork with apple is a classic fall flavor combo. When cooked together with squash, the result is a very satisfying meal. Delicata squash is a perfect match for the apple because it can be easily chopped to a similar size, but acorn or butternut squash can be used as well.

2 (4- to 6-ounce) pork chops, bone-in or boneless

¼ cup chopped mixed herbs of choice

1 teaspoon sea salt

3 tablespoons extra-virgin olive oil, divided

1 leek, cut into ¼-inch slices

1 small delicata, acorn, or butternut, halved, seeded, and cut into half-moons

2 apples, such as Braeburn or Honeycrisp, cored and thinly sliced

¼ cup Bone Broth (page 128)

2 garlic cloves, minced

1. Preheat the oven to 375°F.

2. Coat the pork chops with the herbs and salt. In a large bowl, toss together 1 tablespoon of oil with the leek, squash, and apples.

3. In an ovenproof skillet over medium-high heat, warm 1 tablespoon of oil until sizzling hot. Add the pork chops and cook for 4 minutes per side, until golden-brown. Transfer to a plate.

4. Pour the remaining 1 tablespoon of oil into the skillet and add the apple mixture. Cook, stirring frequently, for 2 minutes. Add the broth and garlic, scraping to deglaze the pan. Cook for 4 minutes, until the liquid has mostly evaporated.

5. Nestle the pork into the skillet, then bake for about 6 minutes or until the pork registers 145°F on an instant-read thermometer and the vegetables are soft. Serve.

PER SERVING: Calories: 541; Total fat: 25g; Carbohydrates: 55g; Fiber: 9g; Protein: 29g; Sodium: 1,244mg

PASTA BOLOGNESE

COMFORT FOOD **WORTH THE WAIT**

Serves 2 / **Prep time:** 15 minutes / **Cook time:** 1 hour 45 minutes

What makes pasta Bolognese special is also what makes it an ideal dish to support gut healing and health: Its slowly braised sauce extracts and retains all the nutrients. This sauce also incorporates liver, which is a powerful source of vitamins essential for healing and rebuilding.

2 ounces uncured/
nitrate-free pancetta or
bacon slices, chopped

1 onion, chopped

1 carrot, chopped

1 celery stalk, chopped

4 garlic cloves, chopped

5 tablespoons extra-virgin
olive oil

4 ounces ground
pasture-raised pork

4 ounces ground grass-fed
beef

3 ounces grass-fed chicken
or beef liver, trimmed and
finely chopped

2 tablespoons balsamic
vinegar

¼ cup Bone Broth
(page 128)

1 cup No-Mato Sauce
(page 122)

1. In a food processor, pulse the pancetta, onion, carrot, celery, and garlic until minced.

2. Heat the oil in a large saucepan over medium heat. Add the pancetta mixture and cook for 5 to 6 minutes, until the pancetta begins to brown and the onion is translucent and browning.

3. Add the pork, beef, and liver to the pan, and cook for 3 to 5 minutes, stirring occasionally with a wooden spoon to break up the meat. Add the vinegar and broth to deglaze the pan, then cook for 3 minutes or until reduced by half.

4. Add the no-mato sauce, bay leaves, parsley, oregano, thyme, and 1 teaspoon of salt and bring to a simmer. Reduce the heat to low, cover, and cook for 70 to 90 minutes, until the color is deep and there is almost no liquid. Taste and add salt as needed.

5. About 20 minutes before the sauce is done, bring a large stockpot of water to a boil. Add the remaining 2 tablespoons of salt. Add the pasta and cook according to the package instructions, usually about 10 minutes. Drain.

2 bay leaves

1 tablespoon chopped fresh parsley

1 teaspoon dried oregano

½ teaspoon dried thyme

1 teaspoon sea salt, plus 2 tablespoons

½ (14-ounce) package cassava pasta, such as spaghetti or tagliatelle

6. Remove the bay leaves from the sauce. Serve the pasta in a bowl with a generous amount of sauce ladled over the top. Store leftover sauce in the refrigerator.

MAKE-AHEAD TIP: Make the sauce up to 3 days in advance to have a quick meal ready to go.

PER SERVING: Calories: 1,212; Total fat: 71g; Carbohydrates: 100g; Fiber: 9g; Protein: 42g; Sodium: 8,718mg

LAMB ROAST WITH GOLDEN BEETS

WORTH THE WAIT

Serves 6 to 8 / **Prep time:** 15 minutes / **Cook time:** 4 hours 20 minutes

Lamb roast might feel like a splurge, but you can get a lot of meals out of a three-pound shoulder, and it is packed with iron and B_{12}. The roasted golden beets and shallots make a perfect fall accompaniment to the richness of the lamb.

½ cup extra-virgin olive oil

4 garlic cloves, mashed or grated

¼ cup mixed herbs of choice

1 (3-pound) boneless lamb shoulder, trimmed of visible fat

4 to 6 golden beets, quartered

6 shallots

1 garlic bulb, top chopped off and soaked with olive oil

1 cup Bone Broth (page 128)

1 teaspoon sea salt

1. Preheat the oven to 450°F.

2. In a small bowl, whisk together the oil, garlic, and herbs. Spread half the oil mixture on the lamb. Heat a large skillet over medium-high heat. Sear the lamb on all sides, about 1 minute. Transfer to a roasting pan.

3. In a large bowl, toss the beets, shallots, and garlic bulb with the remaining oil mixture. Transfer the vegetables to the roasting pan. Roast for 20 minutes, then turn the heat down to 300°F and cook for 3 to 4 hours, until the lamb registers 180°F on an instant-read thermometer and the vegetables are tender.

4. Transfer the vegetables to a serving dish. Squeeze out the garlic cloves and mix together. Break up the lamb by slicing or shredding, then arrange it on top of the roasted vegetables. Serve.

MAKE-AHEAD TIP: Because the roast is large, it works well to cook this on the weekend and have leftovers for the week. If you want to speed up the process, cube the shoulder and cook in the pressure cooker for 50 minutes. Serve it like pulled pork.

PER SERVING: Calories: 535; Total fat: 34g; Carbohydrates: 10g; Fiber: 2g; Protein: 48g; Sodium: 584mg

MEATBALLS WITH FAUX-PEANUT SAUCE AND GREENS

30 MINUTES OR LESS   ONE-POT MEAL

Serves 4 / **Prep time:** 10 minutes / **Cook time:** 15 minutes

This Thai-style faux–peanut sauce uses tigernut flour to mimic the peanut butter normally used. If the sauce isn't thickening, add more tigernut a teaspoon at a time and give it a minute to thicken.

1 pound ground grass-fed beef

4 garlic cloves, chopped, divided

1 teaspoon dried lemongrass

½ teaspoon sea salt

3 tablespoons avocado or coconut oil, divided

1 bunch spinach or rainbow chard, thinly sliced

Sea salt

2 tablespoons coconut aminos, divided

½ teaspoon ground ginger

2 shallots, thinly sliced

½ (14-ounce) can coconut milk (no gums or carrageenan)

3 tablespoons tigernut flour

2 tablespoons chopped fresh cilantro

. . . .

PER SERVING: Calories: 463; Total fat: 35g; Carbohydrates: 12g; Fiber: 3g; Protein: 26g; Sodium: 579mg

1. Preheat the oven to 350°F.

2. In a large bowl, mix together the beef, half the garlic, the lemongrass, and the salt. Form into 14 to 16 meatballs.

3. In a wok or large skillet over medium-high heat, warm 1 tablespoon of oil. Add the meatballs and cook for about 4 minutes, browning on all sides. Transfer them to an oven-safe pan and keep warm in the oven.

4. Clean out the wok and return it to medium-high heat with 1 tablespoon of oil. Add the spinach, a pinch of salt, and 1 tablespoon of coconut aminos. Cook, stirring frequently, for about 2 minutes, until the spinach wilts. Transfer to the pan in the oven.

5. Clean out the wok and return it to medium-high heat with the remaining 1 tablespoon of oil and the remaining 1 tablespoon of coconut aminos. Add the remaining half of the garlic, the ginger, and the shallots. Cook for 1 minute, then add the coconut milk. Bring to a strong simmer, then whisk in the tigernut flour and cilantro until combined. Season with salt. Reduce the heat and cook for 2 to 3 minutes, until thickened.

6. Remove the meatballs and spinach from the oven. Serve the greens as a bed for the meatballs and cover them with sauce.

LAMB BURGERS WITH SPINACH SALAD

30 MINUTES OR LESS

Serves 2 / **Prep time:** 5 minutes / **Cook time:** 10 minutes

Lamb has more iron than chicken or fish and is loaded with B vitamins. We added enough yogurt-mint dressing in this recipe to cover the salad and the burger.

FOR THE LAMB BURGERS

8 ounces ground pasture-raised lamb

1 garlic clove, minced

½ teaspoon chopped fresh mint

½ teaspoon chopped fresh oregano

½ teaspoon chopped fresh dill

½ teaspoon sea salt

1 teaspoon avocado oil

FOR THE SPINACH SALAD

3 tablespoons extra-virgin olive oil

¼ cup Coconut Yogurt (page 121)

Juice of ½ lemon

Sea salt

1 teaspoon chopped fresh mint

1½ cups baby spinach

½ English cucumber, diced

¼ red onion, thinly sliced

¼ cup kalamata olives, pitted

TO MAKE THE LAMB BURGERS

1. In a large bowl, combine the lamb, garlic, mint, oregano, dill, and salt. Form into 2 patties.

2. In a large skillet over medium-high heat, warm the oil. Add the patties and cook for 4 minutes, then flip and cook for about 4 more minutes or until the burgers register 150°F on an instant-read thermometer.

TO MAKE THE SPINACH SALAD

3. In a small bowl, whisk together the oil, yogurt, lemon juice, a pinch of salt, and the mint until emulsified.

4. Arrange the spinach on two plates with the cucumber, onion, and olives. Top with the burgers and pour the yogurt dressing over everything. Serve.

PER SERVING: Calories: 608; Total fat: 53g; Carbohydrates: 7g; Fiber: 2g; Protein: 28g; Sodium: 995mg

BROCCOLI BEEF STIR-FRY

30 MINUTES OR LESS   ONE-POT MEAL

Serves 4 / **Prep time:** 10 minutes / **Cook time:** 10 minutes

If you have a craving for takeout, this broccoli beef dish will hit the spot. Serve with cauliflower or cassava rice. Add a cup of Bone Broth warmed with coconut aminos, salt, and scallions for a quick side of soup.

¼ cup Bone Broth
(page 128)

¼ cup coconut aminos

1 tablespoon tapioca starch

1 tablespoon honey

2 teaspoons minced garlic

2 teaspoons minced fresh
ginger

2 tablespoons avocado or
coconut oil, divided

1 pound flank steak, skirt
or sirloin tip, thinly sliced
across the grain

½ onion, cut into thin
wedges

2 cups broccoli florets,
blanched in salted water

2 teaspoons scallion, white
parts only, cut on the bias

Sea salt

Cauliflower or cassava rice,
for serving

1. In a medium bowl, whisk together the broth, coconut aminos, tapioca starch, honey, garlic, and ginger. Set aside.

2. In a wok or large skillet over high heat, warm 1 tablespoon of oil, swirling to coat the pan, until sizzling hot. Add the beef and stir-fry for 3 minutes, until just cooked through. Set aside on a plate.

3. Rinse and dry the wok and return to high heat with the remaining 1 tablespoon of oil. Add the onion, broccoli, and scallion, and stir-fry for 2 minutes. Add the reserved beef. Pour in the sauce and bring to a boil. Reduce the heat to low and cook for about 2 minutes, until thickened.

4. Taste and add salt as needed. Serve over cauliflower rice.

PER SERVING: Calories: 324; Total fat: 17g; Carbohydrates: 13g; Fiber: 2g; Protein: 26g; Sodium: 349mg

MEATLOAF WITH CELERIAC MASH

COMFORT FOOD **WORTH THE WAIT**

Serves 6 / **Prep time:** 15 minutes / **Cook time:** 1 hour

Using more than one kind of meat and using vegetables for a third of the loaf makes for a moist, flavorful meatloaf. This version is a family favorite.

FOR THE MEATLOAF

3 tablespoons extra-virgin olive oil, divided

4 garlic cloves, chopped

3 celery stalks, chopped

2 carrots, chopped

1 onion, chopped

1½ teaspoons sea salt, divided

1 pound ground grass-fed beef

½ pound ground pasture-raised pork or turkey

1 tablespoon pasture-raised gelatin, bloomed in 1 tablespoon of water

1 tablespoon chopped fresh parsley

2 teaspoons dried oregano

1 teaspoon dried thyme

TO MAKE THE MEATLOAF

1. Preheat the oven to 400°F. Line a rimmed baking sheet with aluminum foil.

2. In a large skillet over medium heat, warm 1 tablespoon of oil. Add the garlic, celery, carrots, onion, and ½ teaspoon of salt and cook for 7 to 9 minutes, until the vegetables are soft. Remove from the heat and let cool. Transfer to a food processor and pulse, scraping down the sides as needed, until fairly smooth.

3. Transfer the processed veggies to a large bowl. Add the beef, pork, bloomed gelatin, parsley, oregano, thyme, and the remaining 1 teaspoon of salt. Mix thoroughly by hand, then transfer the meat mixture to a glass loaf pan, smoothing out the top. Place on the prepared baking sheet and bake for 30 minutes, until the meatloaf is partially set and slides easily from the pan.

4. Flip the loaf pan over onto the baking sheet and remove, exposing the meatloaf. Brush the loaf with the remaining 2 tablespoons of oil. Bake for another 20 minutes or until the meatloaf registers 165°F on an instant-read thermometer. Remove and let sit, covered, for 10 minutes.

FOR THE
CELERIAC MASH

2 pounds celeriac, cubed

6 tablespoons extra-virgin olive oil

2 garlic cloves, minced

1 shallot, minced

½ teaspoon sea salt, plus more as needed

TO MAKE THE CELERIAC MASH

5. Meanwhile, bring a large pot of water to a boil over high heat. Add the celeriac and cook for about 7 minutes, until soft. Use a slotted spoon to transfer to a large bowl, then drain the pot.

6. Add the oil, garlic, shallot, and salt, mashing it thoroughly. Return to the pot and set over low heat to reduce some of the water. Season with salt to taste.

7. Cut the meatloaf into thick slices and serve with the celeriac mash.

PER SERVING: Calories: 525; Total fat: 39g; Carbohydrates: 20g; Fiber: 4g; Protein: 26g; Sodium: 1,042mg

CARNITAS ON PLANTAIN TORTILLAS

WORTH THE WAIT

Serves 6 to 8 / **Prep time:** 15 minutes / **Cook time:** 1 hour

---

Carnitas is a Mexican pulled pork cooked with some herbs and citrus. It's best to crisp carnitas in a pan before serving, but it's also delicious when eaten soft right out of the pressure cooker.

FOR THE PORK

1 (3-pound) boneless pork butt (shoulder), cut into large cubes

2 teaspoons sea salt

2 tablespoons dried oregano

2 tablespoons minced fresh cilantro

½ teaspoon ground cinnamon

1 teaspoon avocado oil

1 onion, diced

6 garlic cloves, chopped

1 cup Bone Broth (page 128)

Juice of 1 orange or lime

FOR THE TORTILLAS

1 green plantain, chopped

2 tablespoons whole cassava flour, plus more for shaping

Pinch sea salt

TO MAKE THE PORK

1. In a medium bowl, combine the pork, salt, oregano, cilantro, and cinnamon, and mix well.

2. In the pot of an electric pressure cooker on the sauté setting, warm the oil. Add the onion and cook, stirring, for about 2 minutes, until translucent. Add the garlic and cook for about 15 seconds, until fragrant. Add the pork and cook, stirring, for 1 minute, until browning on all sides. Add the broth and orange juice.

3. Select high pressure and cook for 50 minutes. Naturally release the pressure, usually about 10 minutes. Use a fork to twist and shred the pork chunks. If they don't easily shred, pressure cook for another 10 minutes.

TO MAKE THE TORTILLAS

4. Meanwhile, bring a small pot of water to a boil over high heat. Add the plantain and cook for 15 minutes, until soft. Transfer the plantain to a food processor. Add the cassava flour and salt, then process until a soft but tacky dough ball forms.

5. Flour your hands and divide the dough into 6 equal balls. Place one dough ball between two lightly oiled sheets of parchment paper and gently start to press it down with your hands, creating a circle of dough underneath. Use a rolling pin to roll out a 5-inch tortilla about ⅛-inch thick. Leave it between the parchment paper sheets and set aside. Repeat with the remaining dough balls.

6. Heat a large cast-iron skillet over medium heat. Working with one tortilla at a time, peel off one side of the parchment and flip the tortilla over to lay the uncovered side in the skillet. Cook for 1 to 2 minutes, remove the top parchment, and flip, then cook for 1 to 2 more minutes, until brown blisters form. Set aside. Repeat with the remaining tortillas.

7. Set the same skillet over medium-high heat. Add the pork and a ladleful of cooking liquid. Cook until the pork browns on the bottom, 3 to 5 minutes. Serve stuffed in a plantain tortilla.

MAKE-AHEAD TIP: Cook the pulled pork without a pressure cooker, covered in a roasting pan (or in a slow cooker). Bring half the amount of liquid to a simmer, add to the pan, and cook in a 250°F oven for 6 to 9 hours.

PER SERVING: Calories: 591; Total fat: 37g; Carbohydrates: 23g; Fiber: 2g; Protein: 40g; Sodium: 934mg

CUBAN-STYLE PICADILLO WITH FRIED PLANTAINS

COMFORT FOOD

Serves 4 / **Prep time:** 10 minutes / **Cook time:** 25 minutes

Our No-Mato Sauce replaces the tomato in this Cuban-style picadillo. You'll hardly notice the difference as the filling's sweet, sour, and salty flavors perfectly pair with the fried plantains.

3 tablespoons extra-virgin olive oil

1 onion, diced

1 carrot, diced

6 garlic cloves, finely chopped

1 pound ground grass-fed beef

1 white sweet potato, diced

1 cup No-Mato Sauce (page 122)

½ cup Bone Broth (page 128)

1 tablespoon apple cider vinegar

½ cup green olives, pitted

¼ cup raisins

¼ cup capers

½ teaspoon sea salt, plus more as needed

1 cup coconut or avocado oil

2 green plantains, cut into 1-inch rounds

1. Heat the olive oil in a skillet over medium heat. Add the onion and carrot and cook for about 2 minutes, until the onion is translucent. Add the garlic and cook until fragrant, about 15 seconds. Add the beef and cook, stirring frequently to break it up, for 3 to 5 minutes, until browned.

2. Add the sweet potato and cook for about 5 minutes. Add the no-mato sauce, broth, and vinegar, and bring to a simmer. Cook for 5 minutes or until reduced by a third.

3. Reduce the heat to low and add the olives, raisins, and capers. Cook for 5 minutes or until the sweet potato is tender when pierced with a knife. Add the salt, taste, and add more as needed.

4. Meanwhile, in a medium skillet over medium heat, warm the coconut oil. Add the plantains and cook for about 4 minutes per side. They should bubble slightly while cooking but not deep-fry. Transfer to a paper towel–lined plate, then use the bottom of a glass to gently smash each piece until flattened but not breaking apart.

5. Increase the heat to medium-high and heat the oil to 375°F. Add the plantain pieces and cook for 1 minute per side, until browned and crisp on the edges. Use a slotted spoon to transfer them back to the plate. Sprinkle with salt.

6. Serve the picadillo on a plate with the plantains on the side.

PER SERVING: Calories: 792; Total fat: 42g; Carbohydrates: 76g; Fiber: 7g; Protein: 28g; Sodium: 1,205mg

PULLED PORK WITH CASSAVA FRIES

WORTH THE WAIT

Serves 6 to 8 / **Prep time:** 15 minutes / **Cook time:** 1 hour 10 minutes

An electric pressure cooker makes pulled pork easily doable at home. It comes out perfectly every time and is ready in about one (hands-off) hour.

1 (3-pound) boneless pork butt (shoulder), cut into large cubes

3½ teaspoons sea salt, divided, plus more as needed

3 tablespoons avocado oil, divided

1 onion, diced

6 garlic cloves, chopped

1 cup Barbecue Sauce (page 123), divided

1 cup Bone Broth (page 128)

1 cassava, cut into ½-inch-thick planks, then cut again lengthwise

. . . .

PER SERVING: Calories: 731; Total fat: 47g; Carbohydrates: 35g; Fiber: 2g; Protein: 41g; Sodium: 1,823mg

1. Season the pork with 2 teaspoons of salt. In the pot of an electric pressure cooker on the sauté setting, warm 1 tablespoon of oil. Add the onion and cook, stirring, for 2 minutes, until translucent. Add the garlic and cook until fragrant, about 15 seconds. Add the pork and cook, stirring, for about 4 minutes, until browned on all sides.

2. Add ½ cup of barbecue sauce and the broth. Select high pressure and cook for 50 minutes. Naturally release the pressure, usually about 10 minutes. Use a fork to twist and shred the pork chunks. If they don't easily shred, pressure cook for another 10 minutes.

3. Meanwhile, preheat the oven to 500°F on convection setting, if available. Line a rimmed baking sheet with parchment paper.

4. In a large bowl, toss together the cassava, the remaining 2 tablespoons of oil, and the remaining 1½ teaspoons of salt. Arrange the cassava on the prepared sheet with lots of space between the pieces.

5. When the pork is done, bake the cassava for 10 minutes, then flip and cook for 5 minutes more or until tender and browned around the edges. Remove and season with salt.

6. Add the remaining ½ cup of barbecue sauce to the pork and, if needed, some of the liquid. Serve with the cassava fries.

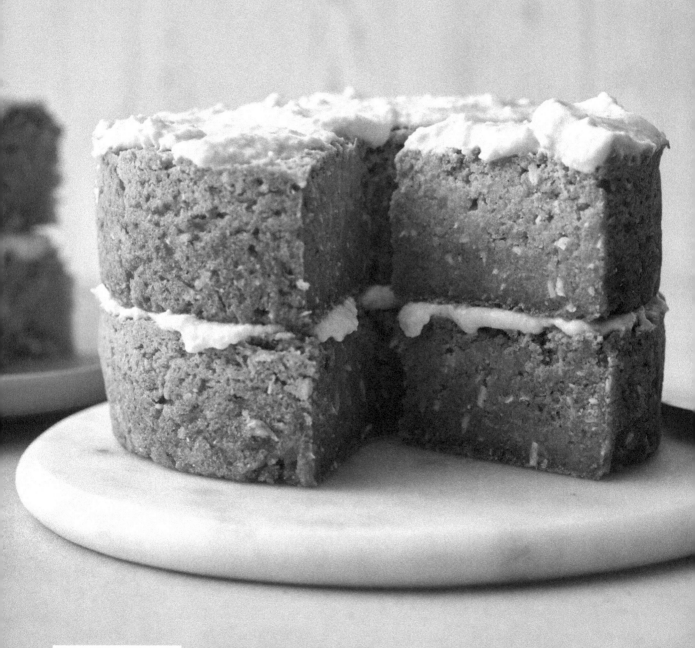

Carrot Cake, *page 113*

CHAPTER 8

SNACKS AND DESSERTS

SARDINES AND TAPENADE ON TOAST

30 MINUTES OR LESS **ONE-POT MEAL**

Serves 2 / **Prep time:** 5 minutes

Packed with omega-3s, calcium, and vitamin D, sardines and mackerel should be on your weekly AIP menu. Tapenade is a tasty accompaniment and condiment. Olives are a great source of healthy fats and are also an easy way to get the electrolyte minerals you need daily.

1 garlic clove, chopped

1 (7-ounce) jar pitted black olives (no preservatives)

1 shallot, chopped

1 tablespoon mixed dried thyme and oregano

1 teaspoon freshly squeezed lemon juice

¼ cup extra-virgin olive oil, plus more as needed

¼ teaspoon sea salt

4 slices AIP Bread (page 129), toasted

Arugula, for serving

1 tin wild sardines or mackerel in olive oil

1. In a food processor, pulse the garlic, olives, shallot, herbs, and lemon juice until minced. Scrape down the sides and add the oil. Pulse until the tapenade becomes a spreadable paste. Season with the salt. Add oil as needed to get the desired texture.

2. Spread the tapenade on the toast, then top with some arugula and sardines and enjoy.

MAKE-AHEAD TIP: Double the tapenade recipe and keep it in a glass jar in the refrigerator. It will keep for up to a month if covered with a layer of olive oil.

PER SERVING: Calories: 713; Total fat: 56g; Carbohydrates: 42g; Fiber: 6g; Protein: 13g; Sodium: 1,818mg

AVOCADO TOAST

30 MINUTES OR LESS **ONE-POT MEAL** **VEGAN**

Serves 2 / **Prep time:** 10 minutes

Avocado is one of the best sources of healthy fats, fiber, vitamins B$_6$ and C, and magnesium. Avocado also goes great on everything from salad to a burger to toast! Scale up the mashed avocado part of the recipe and have dip for cassava tortilla chips, carnitas tacos, or Cuban picadillo.

1 garlic clove, peeled

½ teaspoon sea salt, divided, plus a pinch

½ large avocado, pitted and peeled

Juice of ½ lime

1 shallot, minced

1 tablespoon minced fresh cilantro

4 slices AIP Bread (page 129), toasted

1. Use the back of a knife to mince and mash the garlic with a pinch of salt to form a paste. Transfer to a medium bowl.

2. Add the avocado, lime juice, shallot, cilantro, and ¼ teaspoon of salt. Mash with the back of a fork until well combined and slightly chunky. Season to taste with the remaining ¼ teaspoon of salt.

3. Spread liberally on the toasted bread and serve.

INGREDIENT TIP: Once cut open, avocado browns quickly. To buy yourself some time, cover the cut surface completely with a thin layer of avocado oil and keep in an airtight container. If there is a layer of brown, just scrape it off until you reach the green, and enjoy.

. . . .

PER SERVING: Calories: 324; Total fat: 17g; Carbohydrates: 40g; Fiber: 7g; Protein: 5g; Sodium: 1,209mg

TIGERNUT GRANOLA

5 INGREDIENT   WORTH THE WAIT   VEGAN

Serves 6 / **Prep time:** 5 minutes, plus overnight to soak / **Cook time:** 30 minutes

One of the textures often missed on the AIP diet is crunchy. This granola gives you that crunch, either as a great snack on top of Coconut Yogurt (page 121) or as a topping on ice cream or Apple Crisp (page 111). Tigernuts are not nuts but tubers that are full of prebiotic fiber and good fats.

1 cup whole tigernuts

½ cup large coconut flakes

1 tablespoon maple syrup

1 teaspoon avocado oil or coconut oil, melted

¼ cup dried blueberries, tart cherries, or cranberries, with no additives (optional)

1. Soak the tigernuts overnight in a bowl of water.

2. The next day, preheat the oven to 300°F. Line a baking sheet with parchment paper.

3. Drain the tigernuts and pulse them in a food processor to break into smaller pieces. Alternatively, put them in a zip-top bag and smash with a kitchen mallet.

4. In a large bowl, combine the tigernuts, coconut flakes, maple syrup, and oil, tossing to combine. Use a spatula to spread the mixture out on the prepared baking sheet. Bake for 25 to 30 minutes, stirring every 10 minutes, until browned. Remove from the oven and let cool completely.

5. Once cool, break up and add the dried fruit (if using).

MAKE-AHEAD: Store in a dry airtight container (glass jars are ideal) for up to 3 days in the cupboard or 1 week in the refrigerator.

PER ½ CUP SERVING: Calories: 193; Total fat: 12g; Carbohydrates: 20g; Fiber: 7g; Protein: 2g; Sodium: 3mg

GRAIN-FREE SCONES

30 MINUTES OR LESS

Makes 8 scones / **Prep time:** 10 minutes / **Cook time:** 20 minutes

These scones go great with some tea on a Sunday morning or as a grab-and-go snack during the week. Get creative with the recipe by adding blueberries or dried fruit. I also like making savory scones with chives and bacon (leaving the sugar out).

1 cup whole cassava flour

¾ cup arrowroot or tapioca flour

½ cup coconut oil

Juice of 1 lemon

2 tablespoons coconut sugar or maple syrup

2 tablespoons grass-fed/ finished collagen peptides (see Resources, page 140)

1 tablespoon tigernut or green banana flour

2 teaspoons baking powder

Sea salt

¼ cup water

Coconut butter, for serving

1. Preheat the oven to 350°F. Line a baking sheet with parchment paper.

2. In a food processor, pulse the cassava flour, arrowroot flour, oil, lemon juice, coconut sugar, collagen, tigernut flour, baking powder, and a pinch of salt until well mixed. Add the water, a little at a time, until the dough comes together and is slightly tacky.

3. Flour your hands with a bit of cassava flour and transfer the dough to the prepared baking sheet. Bring the dough together in a loose round loaf about 1 inch thick. Cut into 8 wedges and separate them slightly so they bake independently. Bake for 15 to 20 minutes, until the outside is browned slightly and a toothpick can be inserted and removed cleanly.

4. Cool for 10 to 15 minutes, then serve with coconut butter.

INGREDIENT TIP: Add blueberries or dried cranberries.

MAKE-AHEAD TIP: You can make these scones ahead of time, doubling the batch and freezing.

PER SERVING: Calories: 240; Total fat: 14g; Carbohydrates: 28g; Fiber: 2g; Protein: 3g; Sodium: 142mg

APPLESAUCE

5 INGREDIENT COMFORT FOOD VEGAN WORTH THE WAIT
Serves 5 / **Prep time:** 10 minutes / **Cook time:** 45 minutes

Applesauce is Joshua's number one food hack for inflammation. Supplementing with pectin may provide a similar benefit, but eating applesauce made with the skins has shown the ability to reduce inflammation. And it's delicious!

2 pounds mixed apples of choice

½ cup water

2 teaspoons ground cinnamon

1. Core the apples to remove the seeds, then coarsely chop them, leaving the skins on.

2. Combine the apples and water in a large pot and bring to a simmer over high heat. Lower the heat to low and simmer for 30 to 45 minutes, until the apples are very soft and the pectin has broken down. Add the cinnamon and use a food processor, blender, or food mill to blend and break up the skin.

3. Cool and store in a glass jar in the refrigerator for up to 3 weeks.

INGREDIENT TIP: Green apples—such as Granny Smiths—that are slightly less ripe have the highest amount of pectin, so Joshua always adds a couple to the mix. But you can also use a mix of Fuji, Gala, and Honeycrisp to add a bit of sweetness.

MAKE-AHEAD TIP: If you like to preserve food, spend a weekend in the fall canning applesauce to have all winter and spring. Buy 25 pounds of local apples during peak season and fill a cupboard full of jars.

PER SERVING: Calories: 97; Total fat: <1g; Carbohydrates: 26g; Fiber: 5g; Protein: 1g; Sodium: 2mg

APPLE CRISP

COMFORT FOOD   WORTH THE WAIT   VEGAN

Serves 8 / **Prep time:** 10 minutes / **Cook time:** 50 minutes

Fall is time for apples, and this apple crisp served with a scoop of coconut ice cream will be a great treat when the weather turns a bit cooler. Use whatever kind of apples you can get from your local market or, if you prefer a tart crisp, use green apples.

4 cups cored and sliced apples of choice, peeled or unpeeled

Sea salt

¼ cup freshly squeezed orange juice

½ cup coconut sugar

½ cup whole cassava flour

1 teaspoon ground cinnamon

½ teaspoon ground ginger

½ cup coconut oil, refrigerated

1 cup Tigernut Granola (page 108)

1. Preheat the oven to 350°F. Lightly oil a pie pan or baking dish.

2. In a large bowl, combine the apples, a pinch of salt, and the orange juice. In another bowl, combine the sugar, flour, cinnamon, and ginger. Cut the cold oil into small pieces.

3. Put the apples in the prepared pan, spreading them evenly. Sprinkle the flour mixture over the apples and tuck the pieces of coconut oil around the apples.

4. Bake for 45 minutes or until the apples have broken down and are tender. Sprinkle with the granola and bake for 5 more minutes. Remove and serve warm.

INGREDIENT TIP: When stone fruit is in season, replace the apples with peeled and sliced apricots or peaches.

PER SERVING: Calories: 278; Total fat: 14g; Carbohydrates: 35g; Fiber: 4g; Protein: 2g; Sodium: 23mg

COCONUT BLUEBERRY MAPLE ICE CREAM

5 INGREDIENT   **VEGAN OPTION**

Serves 4 / **Prep time:** 10 minutes, plus 4 hours to freeze / **Cook time:** 10 minutes

Homemade ice cream is not as difficult to make as people may think. The job of an ice cream maker is to stir or churn the liquid while it freezes to keep the mixture from creating ice crystals. We can accomplish similar results by stirring the mixture every 30 to 45 minutes, until it becomes too difficult to mix.

2 (12- to 14-ounce) cans coconut milk, or 1 can milk and 1 can cream (no gums or additives)

1 to 2 cups maple syrup

2 scoops grass-fed/ finished collagen peptides (optional, see Resources, page 140)

¼ teaspoon sea salt

1 cup frozen blueberries

1. In a medium saucepan over medium heat, bring the coconut milk, coconut cream, and maple syrup to a simmer. Add the collagen and whisk until fully combined. Add the salt, taste for sweetness, and adjust as needed. Remove from the heat and cool.

2. Transfer the mixture to a freezer-proof container and freeze for 30 to 45 minutes. Remove and stir with a fork or paddle-like spoon and add the blueberries. Return to the freezer and repeat this process two or three times, until it becomes too difficult to stir.

INGREDIENT TIP: Replace the blueberries with chunks of stone fruit or other berries, such as blackberries or raspberries. You can also replace half the liquid with coconut yogurt for a tart frozen yogurt dish instead of ice cream.

PER SERVING: Calories: 556; Total fat: 32g; Carbohydrates: 68g; Fiber: 3g; Protein: 7g; Sodium: 201mg

CARROT CAKE

WORTH THE WAIT

Serves 8 / **Prep time:** 30 minutes, plus 45 minutes to hydrate
Cook time: 50 minutes

The maple syrup and applesauce help keep this cake moist and sweet without being overly sugary. The yogurt glaze replaces the standard cream cheese frosting.

½ cup Coconut Yogurt (page 121)

¼ cup maple syrup, plus ½ cup

½ cup tapioca starch

¼ cup coconut oil, melted, plus more for greasing

2 cups whole cassava flour

1 cup tigernut flour

½ cup unsweetened shredded coconut

1 tablespoon ground cinnamon

1 teaspoon baking soda

½ teaspoon sea salt

¼ teaspoon ground ginger

3 cups carrots, grated

2½ cups coconut milk (no gums or carrageenan)

¼ cup Applesauce (page 110)

1 tablespoon apple cider vinegar

. . . .

PER SERVING: Calories: 391; Total fat: 17g; Carbohydrates: 59g; Fiber: 6g; Protein: 2g; Sodium: 333mg

1. In a small bowl, combine the yogurt, ¼ cup of maple syrup, and the tapioca starch and stir thoroughly. Refrigerate to hydrate. The finished thickness should easily coat the back of a spoon. The longer you can hydrate, the better the glaze will taste (as long as overnight).

2. Preheat the oven to 350°F. Lightly grease two 7-inch cake pans with coconut oil and line the bottoms with rounds of parchment paper cut to fit.

3. In a large bowl, thoroughly combine the cassava and tigernut flours, coconut, cinnamon, baking soda, salt, and ginger. In a separate bowl, combine the carrots, coconut milk, applesauce, vinegar, and the remaining ½ cup of maple syrup. Stir the carrot mixture into the flour mixture, then stir in the oil until a loose dough forms.

4. Evenly divide the batter between the prepared pans, smoothing the tops with a spatula. Bake for 40 to 50 minutes, until a toothpick inserted comes out clean. Remove and cool in the pans for 10 minutes, then transfer to a cooling rack.

5. Pour and spread half the glaze over the top of one cake. Place the second cake on top and pour on the remaining glaze, spreading it to drip over the edge. Slice and serve.

COCONUT SHORTBREAD COOKIES

30 MINUTES OR LESS

Makes 15 cookies / **Prep time:** 20 minutes / **Cook time:** 10 minutes

These coconut shortbread cookies are a delicious small treat, can be made on the fly, and get even better when stored and eaten out of the refrigerator.

½ cup coconut oil

3 tablespoons coconut sugar

¾ cup whole cassava flour

¼ cup arrowroot starch or tapioca flour

¼ cup unsweetened shredded coconut

1 scoop grass-fed/finished collagen peptides (see Resources, page 140)

1 teaspoon baking powder

⅛ teaspoon sea salt

3 tablespoons water

1. Preheat the oven to 350°F. Line a baking sheet with parchment paper.

2. With an electric mixer, beat the oil with the sugar until light and fluffy.

3. In a large bowl, mix together the cassava flour, arrowroot starch, coconut, collagen, baking powder, and salt. Add the flour mixture to the oil-sugar mixture. Add the water and mix to form a slightly sticky dough.

4. Roll the dough into balls, each about 1 tablespoon. Put them on the prepared baking sheet, then press them slightly with the bottom of a jar to a ½-inch thickness.

5. Bake for about 10 minutes, until golden. Cool completely before eating, as they will be crumbly when warm. They will get even better in the refrigerator overnight.

SUBSTITUTION TIP: Replace the coconut sugar with honey or maple syrup, depending on what kind of sweetener you prefer, though you may need to reduce the amount of water if you are using a liquid sweetener.

PER SERVING: Calories: 114; Total fat: 8g; Carbohydrates: 10g; Fiber: 1g; Protein: 1g; Sodium: 61mg

BANANA CREAM WITH COCONUT WHIP

COMFORT FOOD

Serves 6 / **Prep time:** 10 minutes, plus 2 hours to chill / **Cook time:** 10 minutes

This banana cream can be embellished with fresh berries or unsweetened shredded coconut. Be sure to use grass-fed and pasture-raised gelatin to make sure you aren't consuming glyphosate, a common herbicide that often shows up in conventional gelatin packets.

1 (14-ounce) can coconut milk (no gums or carrageenan)

2 tablespoons honey or maple syrup, plus ½ teaspoon

1 tablespoon pasture-raised gelatin, bloomed in 1 tablespoon water, plus ¼ teaspoon

2 ripe bananas, mashed

½ teaspoon ground cinnamon

½ can coconut cream (no gums or additives)

Sea salt

1. In a small saucepan over medium-high heat, bring the coconut milk and 2 tablespoons of honey to just a simmer. Whisk in 1 tablespoon of bloomed gelatin. Remove from the heat.

2. In a food processor or blender, puree the bananas. Add the cinnamon and coconut milk mixture and blend until smooth. Transfer the mixture to one large container or individual ramekins and refrigerate for about 2 hours, until set.

3. In a small saucepan over medium-high heat, bring the coconut cream and the remaining ½ teaspoon of honey to a simmer. Whisk in the remaining ¼ teaspoon of gelatin. Transfer to a stand mixer fitted with the whisk attachment and whisk until cooled and thickened.

4. Serve the banana cream in small bowls or ramekins topped with whipped coconut cream.

INGREDIENT TIP: If you like banana cream with vanilla wafers, try serving this with Coconut Shortbread Cookies (page 114).

PER SERVING: Calories: 233; Total fat: 17g; Carbohydrates: 19g; Fiber: 2g; Protein: 4g; Sodium: 28mg

PUMPKIN PIE

COMFORT FOOD

Serves 8 / **Prep time:** 15 minutes, plus 2 hours 40 minutes to chill
Cook time: 20 minutes

Although you can find no-additive canned pumpkin puree, try to make your own (see the tip). Fresh pumpkin ensures you won't just get a treat but a lot of great nutrients as well. As always, use pasture-raised gelatin.

FOR THE CRUST

½ cup coconut oil, plus more for greasing pie pan

1¼ cups whole cassava flour

¼ cup tigernut or green banana flour

2 teaspoons pasture-raised gelatin, bloomed in 1 tablespoon water

3 to 5 tablespoons ice-cold water

Pinch sea salt

FOR THE FILLING

2 cups pumpkin puree

½ cup coconut milk (no gums or carrageenan)

2 teaspoons pasture-raised gelatin, bloomed in 1 tablespoon water

¼ cup maple syrup

1 teaspoon ground cinnamon

½ teaspoon ground ginger

¼ teaspoon ground cloves

Sea salt

TO MAKE THE CRUST

1. Preheat the oven to 375°F. Lightly grease a pie pan with coconut oil.

2. In a food processor, combine the cassava flour, tigernut flour, oil, gelatin, 3 tablespoons of water, and the salt. Pulse, adding a bit of water as needed, until the dough comes together in a ball. Remove the dough, place it between two sheets of parchment paper, and roll it out until it is half an inch bigger than the pie pan. Transfer the dough to the prepared pan, fixing any cracks with the bottom of a jar or glass. Refrigerate for 30 to 40 minutes.

3. Lightly poke the crust with a fork and bake until the dough looks dry and slightly browned, 15 to 20 minutes. Set aside to cool.

TO MAKE THE FILLING

4. In a medium saucepan over medium heat, warm the pumpkin puree. Pour the coconut milk into a separate small saucepan over medium heat. Just before the coconut milk simmers, whisk in the bloomed gelatin and stir until fully combined. Remove from the heat.

5. Add the maple syrup, cinnamon, ginger, cloves, and a pinch of salt to the pumpkin puree. Cook for 3 to 5 minutes, until the flavors meld. Pour in the coconut milk mixture and mix thoroughly. Taste and add maple syrup and spices as needed.

6. Pour the filling into the piecrust and refrigerate for 1 to 2 hours, until fully set. Slice and serve.

INGREDIENT TIP: Make pumpkin puree by steaming or roasting seeded pie pumpkin halves until soft. Scoop out the pulp and puree, then reduce further in a pot to get rid of most of the residual water.

. . . .

PER SERVING: Calories: 288; Total fat: 17g; Carbohydrates: 31g; Fiber: 4g; Protein: 3g; Sodium: 49mg

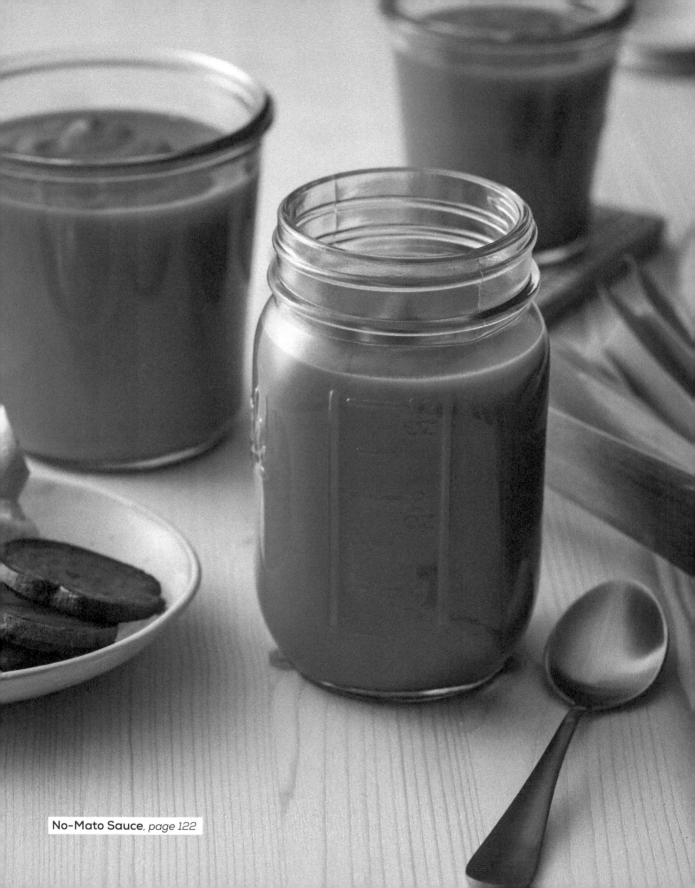

No-Mato Sauce, *page 122*

CHAPTER 9

SAUCES, DRESSINGS, AND STAPLES

BASIL AND SPINACH PESTO

5 INGREDIENT **30 MINUTES OR LESS** **VEGAN**

Makes about 1 cup / **Prep time:** 5 minutes

You can make pesto quickly and use it all week on vegetables, toast, and spaghetti squash. Mix it with oil and balsamic vinegar to make salad dressing. Make the cilantro option (see Substitution tip) to add to the Thai-inspired meals in this book. I frequently have several types of pesto in my refrigerator to give meals a boost with no additional effort.

1 cup fresh basil

½ cup baby spinach

1 teaspoon freshly squeezed lemon juice

2 garlic cloves, peeled

1 tablespoon nutritional yeast

½ teaspoon sea salt

3 to 6 tablespoons extra-virgin olive oil, plus more for preserving

1. In a food processor, combine the basil, spinach, lemon juice, garlic, nutritional yeast, and salt. Pulse until well chopped. Scrape down the sides with a spatula. A little at a time, pour in the oil and blend until smooth, scraping the sides as needed, until all the ingredients come together.

2. Transfer the pesto to an airtight glass container. Cover the top with a layer of oil to prevent the herbs from browning. Store in the refrigerator for up to 1 week.

SUBSTITUTION TIP: To make cilantro pesto, replace the basil, spinach, lemon juice, and olive oil with 1 bunch of cilantro, 1 thinly sliced lemongrass stalk, 1 makrut (kaffir) lime leaf (optional), 1 teaspoon of lime juice, and 3 to 6 tablespoons of avocado oil. Use extra avocado oil to preserve it.

PER BATCH: Calories: 406; Total fat: 41g; Carbohydrates: 6g; Fiber: 2g; Protein: 6g; Sodium: 1,199mg

COCONUT YOGURT

5 INGREDIENT   VEGAN OPTION

Makes about 1 quart / **Prep time:** 10 minutes

Cook time: 5 minutes, plus up to 24 hours to ferment

Homemade yogurt is easy if you have an electric pressure cooker with a yogurt setting. Make your yogurt from a starter culture rather than commercial yogurt—several brands are available. I use a Bifido starter from NPSelection (see Resources, page 140).

2 (14-ounce) cans coconut milk (no gums or carrageenan)

10 grams pasture-raised gelatin, bloomed in ¼ cup water

20 grams tapioca starch

1 sachet yogurt starter culture

INGREDIENT TIP: Yogurt made with dairy thickens as it ferments, but coconut milk must be thickened with gelatin and starch. Too much gelatin makes the texture like a jellied dessert, whereas too much starch makes the yogurt pasty. You can also use agar agar instead of gelatin and look for a nondairy-based starter for a vegan option.

1. Sterilize an electric pressure cooker pot by boiling water in it for 5 minutes, then drain. Pour in the coconut milk, set the cooker to boil or sauté, and cover and seal the cooker, leaving the vent open. Bring to a boil, usually about 5 minutes. Remove the pot from the cooker. Whisk in the bloomed gelatin and starch and let it cool to between 104°F and 110°F.

2. Whisk in the yogurt starter culture, return the pot to the cooker, and select the yogurt setting. Cover and let it ferment for up to 24 hours. The longer the fermentation, the sourer the yogurt. If the yogurt doesn't smell fermented, you likely added the starter when the liquid was too hot, or your starter was dead. You won't have yogurt, but you will have a thickened coconut milk ready for soup or curry.

3. Transfer the yogurt to a sterilized glass jar and refrigerate. Use 2 to 3 tablespoons from this batch to make 2 to 3 additional yogurt batches without the starter.

PER ½ CUP SERVING: Calories: 185; Total fat: 17g; Carbohydrates: 7g; Fiber: 1g; Protein: 3g; Sodium: 17mg

NO-MATO SAUCE

VEGAN OPTION **WORTH THE WAIT**

Makes about 1 quart / **Prep time:** 10 minutes / **Cook time:** 45 minutes

This is a versatile red sauce made without the nightshades. Our No-Mato Sauce keeps the earthiness of the beets in check by punching up the umami with mushrooms, balsamic vinegar, and coconut aminos. Make sure to use no-bone broth if you eat plant-based.

3 golden beets, quartered

1 red beet, quartered

1 cup large cubed butternut squash or chopped carrots

2 cups Bone Broth or no-bone broth (see Substitution tip, page 128)

½ cup cremini mushrooms

½ cup extra-virgin olive oil

1 large leek, sliced

2 tablespoons balsamic vinegar

6 garlic cloves, chopped

½ cup coconut aminos

1 teaspoon sea salt

1. Bring a large pot of water to a boil over high heat. Add the golden and red beets and the squash and cook for 10 to 15 minutes, until the vegetables are soft all the way through. Remove from the pot, let cool slightly, and peel the beets.

2. Meanwhile, in a medium pot over medium-low heat, warm the broth.

3. In a blender, combine the warmed broth, beets, squash, mushrooms, oil, leek, vinegar, garlic, coconut aminos, and salt and blend until completely smooth. Empty into a medium saucepan.

4. Set the saucepan over medium heat and bring to a simmer. Reduce the heat to low and cook for 20 to 30 minutes, until slightly reduced and the color has deepened. Taste and add salt as needed. Store in glass jars in the refrigerator for up to 1 week.

INGREDIENT TIP: To make an Italian-style sauce, add 1 tablespoon of mixed oregano, thyme, and sage.

. . . .

PER CUP: Calories: 375; Total fat: 29g; Carbohydrates: 26g; Fiber: 5g; Protein: 5g; Sodium: 1,203mg

BARBECUE SAUCE

30 MINUTES OR LESS **VEGAN OPTION**

Makes about 1½ cups / **Prep time:** 5 minutes / **Cook time:** 10 minutes

Nothing beats a tangy barbecue sauce. Our sauce uses No-Mato Sauce as the base and adds depth of flavor with molasses, honey, and smoked sea salt. Use whatever form of the sauce you have in the refrigerator; any herbs you've incorporated will add character. Add some horseradish for a bit of heat.

1 teaspoon avocado or extra-virgin olive oil

2 garlic cloves, minced

1 shallot, minced

1 tablespoon unsulfered blackstrap molasses

1 tablespoon maple syrup or honey

1 tablespoon coconut aminos

1 cup No-Mato Sauce (page 122)

½ teaspoon smoked sea salt

1. In a medium saucepan, heat the oil over medium-low heat. Add the garlic and shallot and cook until the shallot is translucent, about 1 minute.

2. Add the molasses, maple syrup, and coconut aminos. Stir to incorporate. Add the no-mato sauce, stir, and bring to a simmer. Cook for 5 minutes. Season with the salt. Store in a glass jar in the refrigerator for up to 1 week.

PER ½ CUP: Calories: 188; Total fat: 11g; Carbohydrates: 20g; Fiber: 2g; Protein: 2g; Sodium: 892mg

TERIYAKI SAUCE

30 MINUTES OR LESS **VEGAN OPTION**

Makes about 1½ cups / **Prep time:** 5 minutes / **Cook time:** 10 minutes

Teriyaki Sauce is great to have on hand to add to fish or chicken and some stir-fried vegetables for a quick meal. Typically made by combining soy with sugar and citrus juice, our sauce gets its umami from our No-Mato Sauce and coconut aminos.

½ cup coconut aminos

½ cup freshly squeezed orange juice

2 tablespoons No-Mato Sauce (page 122)

2 tablespoons maple syrup or honey

2 garlic cloves, minced

1 scallion, green and white parts, minced

1 teaspoon minced fresh ginger

½ teaspoon sea salt

1 teaspoon tapioca or arrowroot starch, dissolved in ¼ cup water

1. In a medium saucepan over medium-low heat, warm the coconut aminos, orange juice, and no-mato sauce. Add the maple syrup, garlic, scallion, and ginger. Stir to incorporate and bring to a simmer.

2. Season with the salt. Stir in the tapioca starch and cook until slightly thickened, 2 to 3 minutes. Remove from the heat and let cool. Store in a glass jar in the refrigerator for up to 1 week.

....

PER ½ CUP: Calories: 119; Total fat: 1g; Carbohydrates: 25g; Fiber: 1g; Protein: 1g; Sodium: 1,163mg

EGGLESS MAYO

5 INGREDIENT   **30 MINUTES OR LESS**

Makes about 1½ cups / **Prep time:** 5 minutes

Mayonnaise is a magic condiment of emulsified fat and protein, typically made with eggs. We mimic this with the help of Coconut Yogurt, which has starch and gelatin, and by adding some collagen peptides and lemon juice to complete the tangy flavor profile.

½ cup Coconut Yogurt
(page 121)

1 teaspoon freshly squeezed
lemon juice

1 scoop grass-fed/finished
collagen peptides (see
Resources, page 140)

¼ teaspoon sea salt

½ cup plus 2 tablespoons
avocado oil

1. In a food processor, combine the yogurt, lemon juice, collagen, and salt, and mix thoroughly. With the machine running, slowly add the oil until fully incorporated. The combination should start oily and begin to thicken. It won't be as thick as traditional mayonnaise, but it will be spreadable.

2. Taste and add salt as needed. Store in a glass jar in the refrigerator for up to 1 week.

INGREDIENT TIP: Use this mayo as a jumping-off point for tartar sauce by adding minced pickle, dill, and coconut aminos. Make a spicy version for Nori Salmon Wraps (page 62) by adding lemon juice and wasabi. Make an aïoli with lemon juice and crushed garlic.

PER 1 TABLESPOON: Calories: 59; Total fat: 7g; Carbohydrates: <1g; Fiber: 0g; Protein: <1g; Sodium: 27mg

ITALIAN VINAIGRETTE

5 INGREDIENT   30 MINUTES OR LESS   VEGAN OPTION

Makes about 1 cup / **Prep time:** 5 minutes

This vinaigrette is a classic tangy, herbed staple to have on hand for dressing up a salad or punching up some leftover chicken or fish for a quick lunch wrap.

1 garlic clove, minced

¼ teaspoon sea salt, plus a pinch and more as needed

½ cup extra-virgin olive oil

¼ cup apple cider vinegar

1 teaspoon maple syrup or honey

1 tablespoon mixed dried herbs, such as oregano, thyme, marjoram, basil

1. Sprinkle the garlic with a pinch of salt and mash with the side of a knife until it becomes a paste.

2. In a small bowl, whisk together the oil, vinegar, and maple syrup until emulsified. Add the garlic paste, herbs, and ¼ teaspoon of salt. Whisk until fully combined.

3. Taste and add more salt as needed. Store in a glass jar in the refrigerator for up to 2 weeks.

. . . .

PER 2 TABLESPOONS: Calories: 125; Total fat: 14g; Carbohydrates: 1g; Fiber: <1g; Protein: <1g; Sodium: 147mg

CREAMY GREEN DRESSING

30 MINUTES OR LESS   VEGAN

Makes about 2 cups / **Prep time:** 5 minutes

This is another great condiment to have on hand for making meals a little more special. This dressing is avocado-based, thick, and creamy.

1 avocado

¼ cup avocado oil

1 garlic clove, peeled

Juice of 1 lemon

½ bunch flat-leaf parsley

4 fresh chives

2 tablespoons nutritional yeast

½ teaspoon sea salt, plus more as needed

Water, as needed

1. In a food processor or blender, combine the avocado, oil, garlic, lemon juice, parsley, chives, nutritional yeast, and salt. Process until fully smooth. If it is too thick, add enough water to get to a slightly thick but pourable dressing.

2. Taste and add salt as needed. Store in a glass jar in the refrigerator for up to 1 week.

PER 2 TABLESPOONS: Calories: 51; Total fat: 5g; Carbohydrates: 2g; Fiber: 1g; Protein: 1g; Sodium: 78mg

BONE BROTH

5 INGREDIENT   VEGAN OPTION   WORTH THE WAIT

Makes about 4 quarts / **Prep time:** 10 minutes / **Cook time:** 16 to 24 hours

Bone Broth should be a go-to food for anyone with Crohn's and IBD. Great bone broth is cooked for a full day, pulling the nutrients and minerals from the bones and breaking down the cartilage into vital collagen (stock is cooked for only an hour or two). The more cartilage in the bones, the better. The apple cider vinegar maximizes the amount of minerals pulled from the bones.

1 pound beef bones, with knuckles (if available) or the bones of a whole chicken

3 to 4 quarts water

1 tablespoon apple cider vinegar

1. If using bones that haven't been roasted, boil water in a large pot and submerge the bones for 2 minutes to remove impurities. Discard the water.

2. Put the bones, water, and vinegar in the pot of an electric pressure cooker. Set to high pressure for as long as the cooker will allow, with the "keep warm" setting on. Cook for 8 hours or more under pressure. The broth can be left on "keep warm" between cycles. Try for 16 to 24 hours total in the pot. Alternatively, cook in a stockpot on the stove by first bringing to a simmer over high heat then cooking on low.

3. Remove the bones. If using large beef bones, reserve to make another batch of broth; otherwise, discard them. Strain the broth through a fine-mesh filter into glass jars and store in the refrigerator for up to 1 week or in the freezer until needed.

SUBSTITUTION TIP: To make vegan no-bone broth, use 1 quartered onion or leek, 4 coarsely chopped celery stalks, 1 cup sliced fresh or soaked dried mushrooms 5 garlic cloves, the reserved cut ends of vegetables like kale or cabbage, and a handful of parsley and cilantro sprigs.

. . . .

PER CUP: Calories: 41; Total fat: 3g; Carbohydrates: 0g; Fiber: 0g; Protein: 4g; Sodium: 8mg

AIP BREAD

WORTH THE WAIT

Serves 10 / **Prep time:** 2 hours / **Cook time:** 45 minutes

Few foods are harder to replace on the AIP than bread. This rustic loaf isn't going to have the same kind of integrity as a proper loaf of bread, but it is delicious and satisfying.

1 cup water

2 tablespoons avocado or extra-virgin olive oil

½ cup steamed and mashed green plantains or cassava

1 tablespoon apple cider vinegar

1 teaspoon baking soda

2 scoops grass-fed/finished collagen peptides (see Resources, page 140)

½ cup whole cassava flour

½ cup tapioca starch

1 cup tigernut flour

1 teaspoon sea salt

1. In a food processor, thoroughly combine the water, oil, plantains, and vinegar. Transfer to a large bowl. In a separate bowl, thoroughly combine the baking soda, collagen, cassava flour, tapioca starch, tigernut flour, and salt.

2. Add the flour mixture to the plantain mixture, stirring well to form a slightly tacky but not wet dough. If it is too wet, add more cassava flour, 1 tablespoon at a time, fully incorporating the addition before adding more. If it is too dry, add water, 1 tablespoon at a time.

3. Cover and let sit for 1 hour, until spongy (but not elastic) and risen slightly (but not doubled).

4. Line a baking sheet with parchment paper. With damp hands, transfer the dough to the prepared pan, tucking the edges under with the sides of your hand to "plump" the round, and smoothing the top with damp hands. Cover with plastic wrap and let sit for 30 minutes.

5. Preheat the oven to 375°F. Score the top of the dough with a sharp knife, then bake for 35 to 45 minutes, until it registers 195°F on an instant-read thermometer.

6. Allow to completely cool before slicing. Store in an airtight container in the refrigerator for up to 7 days.

PER SERVING (1 OF 10): Calories: 139; Total fat: 6g; Carbohydrates: 19g; Fiber: 2g; Protein: 2g; Sodium: 371mg

HOMEMADE SAUERKRAUT

VEGAN   WORTH THE WAIT

Makes about 2 quarts / **Prep time:** 10 minutes, plus up to 2 weeks to ferment

Making sauerkraut is easy to do at home but requires patience and attention to the mixture as it ferments. The results surpass commercially available products and are made from the biome of where you live, which may be better for building good bacteria in your gut.

2 pounds cabbage,
outer leaves removed,
quartered, and cored

2 tablespoons salt (no
iodine or anticaking
agents)

2 cups filtered or distilled
water, plus an additional
2 tablespoons salt
dissolved (if needed)

1. Cut each cabbage quarter into ½-inch slices. Transfer to a large bowl and mix in the salt. Let stand for 1 hour.

2. With your hands, squeeze the cabbage for about 2 minutes to break down cell walls and release water, working until what you pick up releases water like from a sponge.

3. Fill quart-size glass jars with the mixture almost to the top, stuffing as tightly as you can to remove any air pockets but leaving a little space for expansion. Pour in the filtered water. The brine *must* cover the vegetables at *all times* so they don't rot. Stuff a chunk of a root vegetable or an outer cabbage leaf into the jar to hold the cabbage below the brine. Loosely screw the lids onto the jars.

4. Leave at room temperature away from direct sunlight to ferment for 5 days, unscrewing the lids daily to remove pressure from the jar. Taste and see if the flavor suits you. If not, leave to ferment longer, checking and tasting daily and continuing to release pressure daily. It may take up to 2 weeks.

5. Transfer the jar to the refrigerator to considerably slow the fermentation. As always, keep the vegetables submerged and remove any that have discolored because of contact with the air.

6. The most common issue with sauerkraut is a scum or mold that may form on the top of the liquid or vegetables that have had contact with the air. You can carefully scoop and discard it. The vegetables in the brine should taste and smell fine. If for any reason the vegetables in the liquid (or the liquid itself) starts to smell or taste bad, throw it all out.

INGREDIENT TIP: You can ferment shredded Brussels sprouts and well-scrubbed root vegetables in a similar manner. Drinking the juice from your ferment as you near the bottom of the batch is a great tonic for digestive health.

PER ½ CUP: Calories: 14; Total fat: <1g; Carbohydrates: 3g; Fiber: 1g; Protein: 1g; Sodium: 894mg

CASSAVA TORTILLAS

5 INGREDIENT   30 MINUTES OR LESS   VEGAN

Makes 8 tortillas / **Prep time:** 10 minutes / **Cook time:** 10 minutes

Cassava Tortillas can be used to replace the plantain tortillas in the other dishes in the book, but they also make great wraps for quick lunches. Stuff with leftovers or a salad, or spread with guacamole for a quick snack.

1½ cups whole cassava flour, plus more for shaping

Sea salt

1 tablespoon avocado oil, plus more for the pan

½ cup warm water

1. In a large bowl, combine the flour, a pinch of salt, and the oil. Add half the water and incorporate, then continue to add water until you get a dough ball that is soft but a bit tacky.

2. Flour your hands with cassava flour and divide into 8 balls of dough. Place one dough ball between two lightly oiled sheets of parchment paper and gently start to press it down with your hands, creating a circle of dough underneath. Use a rolling pin to roll out a 5-inch tortilla about ⅛ inch thick. Leave it between the parchment paper sheets and set aside. Repeat with the remaining dough balls.

3. Heat a bit of oil in a cast-iron skillet over medium heat. Working with one tortilla at a time, peel off one side of the parchment and flip the tortilla to lay the uncovered side in the skillet. Cook for 1 to 2 minutes, remove the top parchment, and flip, then cook for 1 to 2 minutes, until brown blisters form. Repeat with the remaining tortillas.

MAKE-AHEAD TIP: Double or triple the batch and keep most in the freezer for an easy lunch or dinner. They will thaw quickly.

. . . .

PER SERVING: Calories: 90; Total fat: 2g; Carbohydrates: 18g; Fiber: <1g; Protein: <1g; Sodium: 8mg

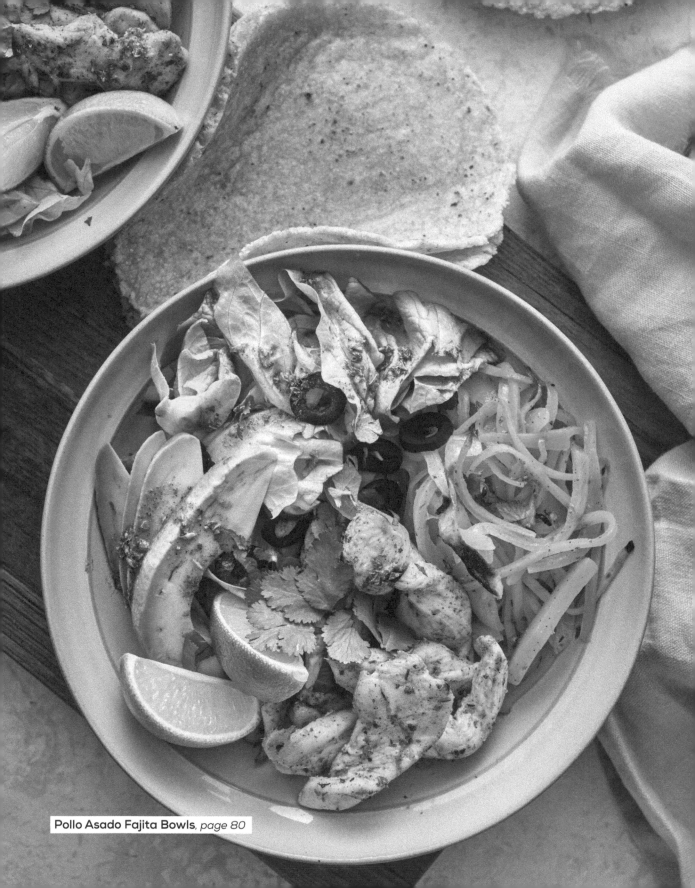

Pollo Asado Fajita Bowls, *page 80*

Measurement Conversions

VOLUME EQUIVALENTS	U.S. STANDARD	U.S. STANDARD (OUNCES)	METRIC (APPROXIMATE)
LIQUID	2 tablespoons	1 fl. oz.	30 mL
	¼ cup	2 fl. oz.	60 mL
	½ cup	4 fl. oz.	120 mL
	1 cup	8 fl. oz.	240 mL
	1½ cups	12 fl. oz.	355 mL
	2 cups or 1 pint	16 fl. oz.	475 mL
	4 cups or 1 quart	32 fl. oz.	1 L
	1 gallon	128 fl. oz.	4 L
DRY	⅛ teaspoon	–	0.5 mL
	¼ teaspoon	–	1 mL
	½ teaspoon	–	2 mL
	¾ teaspoon	–	4 mL
	1 teaspoon	–	5 mL
	1 tablespoon	–	15 mL
	¼ cup	–	59 mL
	⅓ cup	–	79 mL
	½ cup	–	118 mL
	⅔ cup	–	156 mL
	¾ cup	–	177 mL
	1 cup	–	235 mL
	2 cups or 1 pint	–	475 mL
	3 cups	–	700 mL
	4 cups or 1 quart	–	1 L
	½ gallon	–	2 L
	1 gallon	–	4 L

OVEN TEMPERATURES

FAHRENHEIT	CELSIUS (APPROXIMATE)
250°F	120°C
300°F	150°C
325°F	165°C
350°F	180°C
375°F	190°C
400°F	200°C
425°F	220°C
450°F	230°C

WEIGHT EQUIVALENTS

U.S. STANDARD	METRIC (APPROXIMATE)
½ ounce	15 g
1 ounce	30 g
2 ounces	60 g
4 ounces	115 g
8 ounces	225 g
12 ounces	340 g
16 ounces or 1 pound	455 g

How to Reintroduce Foods

After you complete the elimination phase of the autoimmune protocol, it can be both exciting and nerve-racking to start the reintroduction phase. One of the most common questions is this: "How do I know when I can start reintroducing foods?" We recommend that people follow the elimination phase of the protocol for a minimum of 30 days before attempting any reintroductions. On top of that, we want to see that there has been a positive improvement in the management of unwanted symptoms before any eliminated foods are reintroduced to the diet. If you have been following the elimination phase for 30 days and have still not seen the improvements you were hoping for, we recommend following the protocol for another two weeks while also working closely with your health care practitioner to ensure that any potential underlying problems are addressed.

If, after 30 days, you feel that you have seen a positive and dramatic reduction in your most unwanted symptoms, you are likely ready to start the reintroduction phase of the protocol. During the reintroduction phase, it is critical that you proceed with caution—this is not a time to start eating anything and everything. The reintroduction phase is just as strict as the elimination phase and requires just as much planning and dedication, if not more, to execute effectively. This is a time of learning and exploring, when you will discover which foods are your biggest triggers so you can begin to create the most liberal, personalized, anti-inflammatory protocol customized to your own unique needs. During this phase I recommend using a symptom tracker (page 139) to track the foods you have consumed and any associated symptoms. This will allow you to monitor your progress and collect valuable data for your continuing treatment plan.

There are many different ways to approach food reintroduction. The most effective and impactful reintroduction schedule is the longest and most time consuming, but it is also the most likely to yield the best results. This method involves testing a small amount of each new food for three days, and then, if there are no negative reactions, testing a large amount of the new food for three more days. This process is designed to detect both immediate and delayed hypersensitivity reactions, as some foods can cause negative reactions up to 72 hours after consumption. Additionally, many hypersensitivity reactions are dose-related, meaning that a small amount may not produce unwanted symptoms, but a large amount will. In a perfect world, foods should be reintroduced following a schedule like the one set out here (using egg yolk as the example food), which accounts for both delayed reactions and dose-related reactions.

Day 1: Eat a small amount of the untested food—for this example, half a cooked egg yolk.

Days 1 to 3: Monitor your body for two or three days for any unwanted signs and symptoms. If you do not experience any negative reactions, move on to day 4. If you do experience any negative reactions, record them appropriately in your symptom tracker (page 139) and make a note that egg yolks will remain on your eliminated foods list.

Day 4: If you have not experienced a negative reaction since eating the half egg yolk on day 1, now it's time to try a larger test dose—for this example, three cooked egg yolks.

Days 4 to 6: Monitor your body for two or three days for any unwanted signs and symptoms. If you do not experience any negative reactions, continue to enjoy this food in your diet. If you do experience any negative reactions, record them appropriately in your symptom tracker (page 139) and remove the food completely from your diet.

Following this reintroduction method means that a new food will be tested every six days, and we recommend that you only attempt one new food per week. Of course, this is not always feasible. Many people resort to shorter food reintroduction schedules, waiting just one or two days between trials. However, this accelerated method is not ideal because it may make it harder to pinpoint associated symptoms down the road. Ultimately, the best process for you will take into account physical, mental, emotional, and social aspects of real, everyday life. You may even consider working one-on-one with a trained health care professional during this stage of the protocol, because they can offer guidance and draw on their experience to create a unique plan tailored to your lifestyle and symptoms.

Now that we've covered the framework of a food reintroduction schedule, the next step is to determine which foods should be reintroduced first. The following suggested order of food reintroductions was created by the Paleo Mom, Dr. Sarah Ballantyne, based on the likelihood that each food will cause a reaction (in order from least likely to most likely):

1. Egg yolks
2. Grass-fed ghee
3. Seed-derived spices
4. Legumes (except soy)
5. Nuts
6. Seeds
7. Nightshades (except tomatoes)
8. Coffee
9. Chocolate

Of course, this list is not all-encompassing and will be different for each individual. Work with your health care provider to create a customized reintroduction schedule that works best for you and your current situation. At this point, you should continue to avoid gluten, dairy, and soy, as well as any foods you already suspect or know cause sensitivity or allergic reactions. Over time, this process should allow you to create a highly customized anti-inflammatory protocol that is unique to you and your own dietary triggers.

Completing the reintroduction phase as methodically and patiently as possible is the key to ensuring you are getting the most out of the hard work that you put in during the elimination phase of the AIP. The goal is to be able to identify which foods trigger your reactions, eliminate those foods, and enjoy the other foods you know to be "safe" and healthy for your body. Again, the point is not to live on a severely restricted diet forever, but rather to be free from perceived restrictions and enjoy a variety of foods as safely as possible. Having a well-thought-out plan ahead of time is important, and using a symptom tracker (see page 139) is critical for gathering data that will help you create your own customized plan.

Symptom Tracker

Use this page to track symptoms. Make as many copies as you need so you can continue to track symptoms as you reintroduce foods.

DATE	FOOD REINTRODUCED	AMOUNT	SYMPTOMS	DESIGNATION (Okay, Limit, Avoid)

Resources

Some of the ingredients used in this book may be difficult to find at your local grocery store. Try going to a store that specializes in "natural" or organic foods and ask them to stock the items you need. Here are a few other resources:

Amazon.com and **Vitacost.com.** Good resources for specialty flours, such as cassava and tigernut; grass-fed, pasture-raised collagen and gelatin (look for brands like Vital Proteins, Orgain, Dr. Axe Ancient Nutrition, or HVMN); and Bifido yogurt starter. You may also be able to find the high-quality supplements recommended by your nutritionist.

ButcherBox.com. A great resource if you don't have access to grass-fed, organic meats and seafoods locally, and it can save you money with a monthly box delivered to your door.

SeekingHealth.com and **PatchMD.com.** Joshua recommends these sites for supplements and for transdermal (patches) supplementation of nutrients that are difficult to digest and assimilate with Crohn's, such as iron and glutathione. Patches may cause skin irritation in some people. As always, discuss with your nutritionist or health care provider.

References

Jordan, Stefan, Navpreet Tung, Maria Casanova-Acebes, Christie Chang, Claudia Cantoni, Dachuan Zhang, Theresa H. Wirtz, et al. "Dietary Intake Regulates the Circulating Inflammatory Monocyte Pool." *Cell* 178, no. 5 (2019): 1102–1114. doi.org/10.1016/j.cell.2019.07.050.

Konijeti, Gauree G., NaMee Kim, James D. Lewis, Shauna Groven, Anita Chandrasekaran, Sirisha Grandhe, Caroline Diamant, et al. "Efficacy of the Autoimmune Protocol Diet for Inflammatory Bowel Disease." *Inflammatory Bowel Diseases* 23, no. 11 (2017): 2054–2060. doi.org/10.1097/MIB.0000000000001221.

McGonigal, Jane. *SuperBetter*. New York: Penguin Books, 2015.

Sandoval-Ramírez, Berner Andrée, Úrsula Catalán, Lorena Calderón-Pérez, Judit Companys, Laura Pla-Pagà, Iziar A. Ludwig, Ma Paz Romero, and Rosa Solà. "The Effects and Associations of Whole-Apple Intake on Diverse Cardiovascular Risk Factors: A Narrative Review." *Critical Reviews in Food Science and Nutrition* 60, no. 22 (2020): 3862–3875. doi.org/10.1080/10408398.2019.1709801.

Index

About the Authors

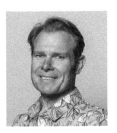

Joshua Bradley is the father and stepfather of four daughters, creator of the Silk Experience fine dining pop-up, and cofounder of NotPie.com and Levered.com. Joshua was diagnosed with Crohn's disease in 2012. After suffering through numerous surgeries and a dysfunctional standard of care, he dove deep into researching genetics, the microbiome, mitochondrial health, tasting, and ketosis. In 2018, Joshua succeeded in reversing his disease state into deep remission and emerged an athlete, competing in two triathlons that year. When he is not in his favorite coffee shop, Joshua spends most of his time reading, cooking, meditating, and running or riding his single-speed bike. You can follow Joshua on Twitter @airjoshb, or on his website GoToStepOne.com.

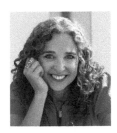

Kia Sanford, MS, holds two master's degrees: one in human clinical nutrition and a second in marriage, family, and child counseling. She uses these in tandem while working with clients to help them foster long-term health. Kia firmly believes that what we eat and drink, and how we move every day, is vitally important, and her understanding that food can be medicine informs her positive focus on all the wonderful things we can eat to create and maintain health. By combining personalized nutrition and psycho-emotional counseling, Kia offers clients a way to understand their present situation and make concrete sustainable changes to move toward sustainable health. Kia's approach works with the many and varied layers of each client, helping create both internal and external environments that are conducive to positive change. You can learn more about Kia at GetRealLifestyle.com.

Printed in the USA
CPSIA information can be obtained
at www.ICGtesting.com
LVHW061949280424
778210LV00002B/5